APPLE, PENNY, CAR

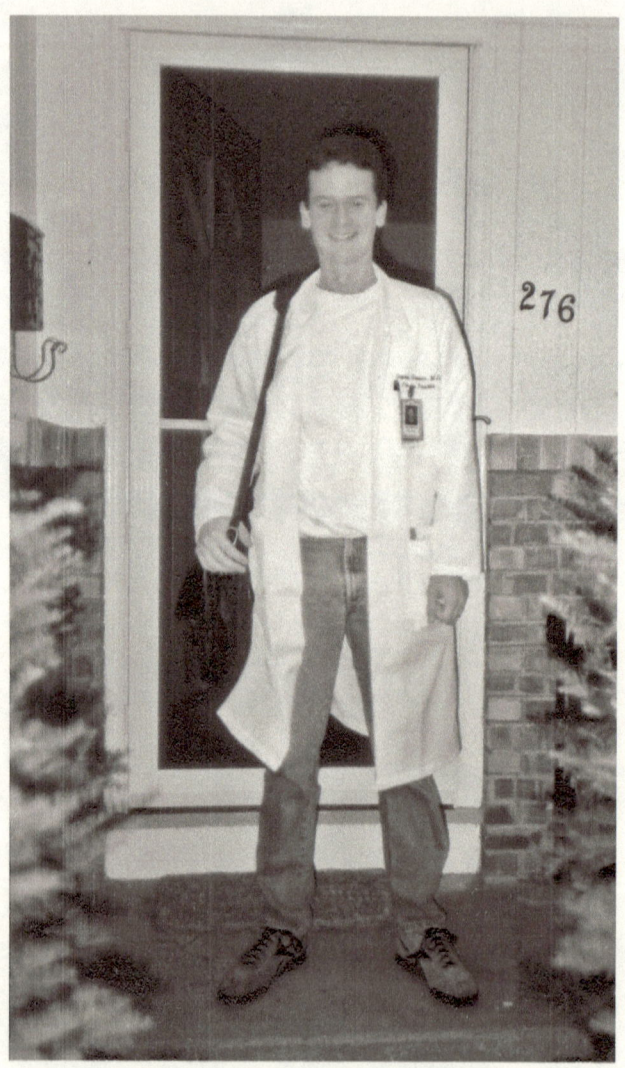

Dan's first day of residency, July 1996.

APPLE, PENNY, CAR

A Doctor's Tale

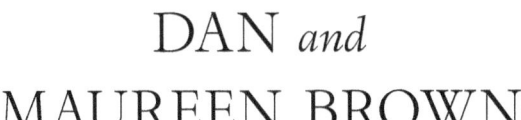

DAN *and*
MAUREEN BROWN

Printed in the United States of America

Designed by Susan Turner

ISBN: 979-8-218-67046-7

RUNNING BANTER BOOKS
SEEKONK, MASSACHUSETTS

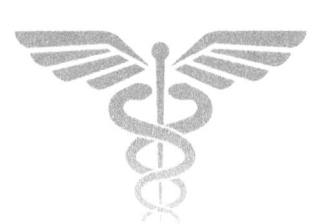

CONTENTS

PREFACE

Maureen

Pick anything in our lives, and you would see that Dan and I have done it together. The journey described in this book is no different. Dan and I grew up in the same little town, half a mile apart. Everyone knew everyone else. Our parents went to school together. Our grandparents worked together. Dan and I formed an unwavering friendship, and by the time we entered high school, we were a bonded pair. Our lives took twists and turns, just like anyone else's—maintaining a long-distance relationship, joyous events, deeply sad losses—but always, in the grand scheme of things, was within the range of normal. This was life, and life was reliably predictable.

Younger-Onset Alzheimer's disease (YOAD), however, was not on the radar. It was almost as if the universe had broken its pact with us. It was a low blow, a red-card-worthy move. It shook us to the core. You can never unknow it. You can never go back to "before." How do you move on from that moment? How do you break that utter paralysis?

It was a slow process. One day, a minute or two of unclenching your jaw. At another time, you share an inside joke that makes you smile, breaking the tension just for a moment. Then there's the day you realize a random thought other than Alzheimer's has entered your consciousness. In fits and starts, we found our feet and, leaning on each other, we started to move through life again.

But we were changed people. We acquired a new barometer for joy, a greater capacity for compassion, and a fine-tuned ability to weed out the drama. We used our medical knowledge to take an emotional break from worrying. The science of it, the rational aspect, was easier to digest. We could deal with it in terms of neurons and plaques and proteins. We relied on our respective roles—Dan as a family physician and me as a neurological occupational therapist—to find our way through this maze of tangles. We managed to start allowing ourselves to see the humor in life again. We relied on each other to try not to be sad all the time.

We needed a way to process everything that happened to us. This book became the embodiment of making good from bad. What better way to continue to teach and help others than to share our story together?

For Dan, lessons from doctoring proved to be a primer in how to treat and be treated. As an occupational therapist (OT), my perspective on ways to live with a neurodegenerative disease helped us focus on hope and meaningful priorities. Could we make living with this disease more tolerable? Less scary? Could we give some boots-on-the-ground intel that would help families anticipate issues rather than feel like every day is a five-alarm fire? Might our story give someone permission to laugh again, despite feeling every emotion but happiness? We had to try.

Dan's kindness and humor were the traits that drew me to him in the first place. His compassion, tenacity, and smarts have made him a physician like few others. Dan has always been a teacher, and his condition has given him a unique perspective on best practices for patient care, priorities for those being treated for a neurodegenerative disease, and living with the disease on a day-to-day basis.

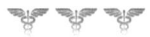

Dan

I have Alzheimer's. When Maureen and I started dating so long ago, I thought, "She is the kindest person I've ever met." And that worked out well because we find fun any way we can, because we laugh, and because I need her. My life has taken some unexpected turns and there have been some rough times. Everything turned upside down when I learned about my condition. It was nothing either of us could have predicted.

Despite that, we are lucky in all sorts of ways. We have a strong community which supports us. We have exceptionally kind family and friends—people who quite literally come running to help us, people who travel cross-country to see us. My family doc asks for my medical opinion when we are weighing health decisions. He has treated me with dignity and compassion and has never failed to be there for me. The team treating my condition is respectful, collaborative, and always ready to think outside the box.

When I first received my diagnosis, Maureen and I pulled over, stopped the car, and just bawled. I lost my job. I lost the practice. In the end, it was probably a blessing in disguise, because odds are I'd still be working as hard as ever. Eventually I realized I never had to be on call again. (I hated call.) Instead of commuting, we walk every day. Instead of sitting in meetings, we see friends. Instead of writing notes, we wrote this book! I think it's a good trade. As I was coming to terms with this condition, I didn't think I was going to live long. I just wanted to travel, do stuff, be active. I wanted to fit everything in. I thought, "I can just wallow in this diagnosis or I can be thankful for what I have."

Looking back on my career, I could have done with less pressure, with a potentially better work/life balance. Without realizing it, over the course of a decade, every day had become Groundhog Day. Up at 4:00 a.m. Drive to work an hour and a half. Grab a coffee on the way. Turn on the office lights. Lunch at 9:00 a.m. Meetings, meetings, meetings. On the road by noon. Race to the office to see patients for six hours. Write notes. Repeat— unless I'm traveling.

On weekends, I took care of the business end of things and desperately tried to connect with my family. I worried about not seeing my kids, about not being a good dad. I also wanted to be the best doc I could and be there for my employees. I was running until the day I left medicine, my medical practice, and my role as the chief medical officer (CMO) of a national health-care system. I gave 100 percent to everything all the time. And I still felt I could have been doing more. I didn't want to just do what had to be done; I wanted to go above and beyond for others. I would come home and say, "Oh, the kids don't have that. I can get it for them." Now I think back on how much time I missed with my family. That was stupid.

I wanted to write this book because I think we are in a unique situation, me as a physician and Maureen as an occupational therapist. I wondered what the best way would be to use our knowledge and experience to help those with the same condition. I needed to let people know that it continues to be a privilege to care, to be trusted. And, of course, I felt an urge and a duty to leave something behind for my loved ones.

If I could send a message to my patients, it would be the

following: I loved being your doc. I hope I have treated you well. Could I have done more? Were there times when I did not do the best for you? If so, I am sorry.

PART I

Dan

1

In the Beginning

My name is Daniel Brown, which tells you nothing about me except that my parents were less than creative when it came time to fill out the birth certificate. Here are some of the details to fill in the gaps.

I love Monty Python. I think science is cool. I sing in the car. I dated my wife for ten years before we got married. I really do want to help people. I have never fallen asleep in class. I love starting fires. I speed. I drink beer, sometimes to the point of intoxication. I had to apply to medical school twice. I started smoking when I was fourteen years old. My favorite color is gray. I always put the seat down. I try to get at least eight hours of sleep a night. I make a mean meatloaf. I percuss really well. I could say the alphabet at two years old. I love mail. I still watch cartoons. My wife dresses me. I watch TV too often. I don't go to church as often as I should. My checkbook is balanced; my diet is not. I've golfed since I was eight years old and have not improved very much. I have no *accent. I don't play guitar very well. I'm a poor speaker but an excellent listener. I like change. I almost killed myself once. I've never seen* Casablanca. *I've never been west of the Mississippi. I'm anal. Ten years from now I hope I'm on vacation. I am Renaissance man. I am becoming my father. I intend to save lives and I expect my patients to die. The relationship that exists between doctor and patient is truly unique, and the aspect of medicine which I find most attractive. I believe in continuity of care, preventative medicine, and all the other catchphrases that have been used to describe family practice. The most important things in my life are my wife, my family, my friends, a sense of humor, golf, and medicine, in that order. It's sixth on the list, and I hope it always stays there. I intend to be very good at what I do, but not at the expense of what I love.*

I came across my residency application essay when I was cleaning out my office. Almost thirty years have passed since I wrote it. I didn't want to write something boring, a fluffy piece on an experience that I had gone through. I wanted something different. I wanted to be upfront and authentic. This is who I am; take me, knowing all of my faults. I intended for it to stir up conversation, given some of the seemingly controversial facts I included. It served its purpose: I did have a rousing discussion with the residency director, and I ended up matching at my program of choice.

Reading the essay now, I am reassured by the consistency of it; most of the facts still ring true. I feel relieved that the things I held in high importance back then remain constants in my life now.

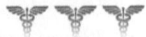

I was a young medical student, and at every turn programs were trying to recruit into their specialties. I was basically a blank slate.

There wasn't much I was averse to trying. Programs would host information nights; the posters were everywhere. I was walking around the medical school one day and saw one that looked interesting. The thing that swayed me to go to the meeting in the end was the promise of free pizza. I was the first person to sign up for the program to learn about family medicine. I was hungry, but I was also intrigued.

An excited and chatty preceptor led the talk and spoke about what family medicine was, what we could expect, what we'd get in return. He promised we would be treating people from all walks of life, and our job, if we were to do it well, was to be ready for everything. "Family medicine provides more care to more people than any other field of medicine," he told us.

In many cases, we could expect to be the doc for our patients through every stage of life. I learned that family medicine had everything I wanted—patients of all age groups, from newborns to the elderly, bringing babies into the world, being present for end of life, consistency of care, and the opportunity to form lifelong relationships with patients. It all came together at that point. I had found my home. At the end of the program, the preceptor told us if we wanted to know more, we could sign up for the shadow program to watch the docs in action. I was hooked. I signed up on the spot and was given a pager, which I loved. I felt like a real doc.

The shadow program gave medical students the chance to "ride along" with the docs. After hours, you might get a page to come to the hospital to meet up with the physician on call. Maybe you would see something interesting that the family doc was called in for, or maybe some other student-friendly physician would be doing something cool, and they would ask you to join them. Some of the best lessons I learned came from these earnest, excited teachers. Over the years, the stories from those experiences became legends. And truth is always stranger than fiction. Some of these stories also mirror events in my life in a way no one could have predicted. It humbles me that I was able to witness these tales. They're too important not to tell.

A NICE GENTLEMAN was being evaluated for cognitive changes using the mini-mental state examination (MMSE), a common test to perform in such cases. Short-term memory is screened by telling the patient three words, then having the patient recall those words after five minutes. When first given the words, our affable patient immediately repeated them back, but he missed every one of them when asked to recall them later. At the end of the session, he asked how he did and was given the bad news that he hadn't done well, having particular trouble on that short-term memory section. He looked dejected and asked, "What were the words?"

"Apple. Penny. Car."

He lowered his head and nodded quietly. We left to see our next patient as he gave us a little wave goodbye.

A week or so later, I joined the attending again on rounds. The nice gentleman was still there and was downright jovial when we entered the room, looking anxious to tell us something. "Hey, Doc," he said, pointing his fingers excitedly at us. "Apple. Penny. Car."

For the entirety of my career, those were the three words I used whenever I completed a mini-mental state exam with a patient. It was a thread that ran through from my first days of medical school through my retirement . . . and beyond.

In another instance during my first year of medical school, my new pager went off with a message from the family doc with the brogue. He let me know he was heading over to the hospital to see a patient. Would I be interested in joining him? I was thrilled and raced on over and met up with him in the emergency department (ED). It turned out not to be as exciting a case as he hoped, but he hooked me up with a giddy surgeon—the tallest person I'd ever seen, incidentally—who was about to place a Foley catheter in a gentleman in preparation for exploratory surgery. He was concerned.

The gentleman was clearly not well. The surgeon chatted the whole time about everything from the proper way to insert the catheter ("firm grasp, pull up, push it in, and release") to best practices for good urinary safety ("never travel in a car with a full bladder"). I was invited to scrub into exploratory surgery for a possible blocked intestine.

Having never been in surgery before, I was briefed on the procedure I'd be dressing into, how to scrub in, and where to stand. The most important rule was not to touch anything. The whole process was surreal. With my blue-gloved hands up in front of me, I elbowed the door open. This was the first time I had ever been in the operating room (OR). It was sparse, efficient, and very bright. Entering the OR is like going into a church sanctuary—few people are allowed the opportunity to enter that space. It was humbling. I was a bit overwhelmed by the situation I had found myself in. I felt the need to whisper.

As I scanned the room, I observed the team gathered around the patient, who was lying on the operating table. He was draped from the waist down with a white hospital sheet, one corner of which was marked in black with the hospital's logo. An unusual set of ramps was set up on either side of the table. The very tall surgeon was there, in addition to another surgeon, who happened to be a little person. The ramp system was built to allow both docs to work easily.

They were so kind. My role: watch, listen, retract, and know when to step back. I was called forward into the sterile space. I couldn't believe what I was witnessing as only a first-year medical student. I actually got blood on my hands. One drop. The surgeons had a relaxed demeanor, but they were earnestly trying to help this guy. Abdominal pain is hard to pinpoint. They were methodical. They proceeded in steps, cutting layer by layer, reporting on what they saw as they went. They initially weren't finding anything suspicious, so they decided to cut a bit deeper into the abdomen. The tall surgeon ran the bowel—inspecting it section by section—and soon announced that he had found a mass. I felt like part of the team. We all were there to witness that moment, a shared experience. As the surgeons teased away the tissues and made an incision in the bowel, we all waited silently. The tall surgeon removed the mass. The whole team cheered. They had found the issue—an intact packet of oyster crackers. Scheming began. They decided to send the specimen to pathology for a full report. Things still excited them. Things still surprised them. My role in this intervention was minor, but it was incredibly meaningful to me. It was a pivotal moment, something that I carried with me my entire career. I got to step behind the curtain, to witness the teamwork, the problem solving, the care, and the passion. The opportunity I was afforded has never been lost on me. It was a great start to my medical career.

I went with two fellow medical students to shadow a physician on the psychiatric ward of the teaching hospital. It's a bit scary to walk onto a locked ward. The whole time we were there, we were at the mercy of the psychiatrist, who had a key. At first glance, the folks on the ward appeared to be acting fairly normal. As I looked closer, I realized some people were indeed wandering about and mumbling to themselves or maybe to someone they envisioned was there alongside them. We weren't given much preparation as to what behaviors we might encounter, but we were encouraged by the doc to interact with folks while we were there. I had put myself into the mindset ahead of the observation to expect the unexpected. One of the conversations I had was with a very pleasant older woman. She was just so kind. I asked her how she was feeling, and she was very positive.

"It's a good day," she said.

"Oh, well, that's great," I replied. "Do you have any children?" I asked. I thought that might be safe terrain.

Again, she was very pleasant. "Oh, yes. I do!"

"Oh, wonderful. How many children do you have?" I asked.

Straight-faced, she replied, "I have 50,000 children." It hit me like a train. Oh wow. It's real.

I tried to steady my voice and not give away my initial surprise. "Oh?" I replied as calmly and pleasantly as I could. I tried to end the conversation quickly and started to make an excuse to leave, but she continued.

"And now you are one of my children too."

She was so pleasant. I was fascinated. It was her truth as she knew it. I felt bad disappointing her and worried about possibly inciting some confusion, so I thought the best approach was to be courteous.

I replied, "Oh, thank you!" She smiled. At that moment, the psychiatrist called us into his office to meet as a team. I said good-bye to the pleasant lady with the many children and went quickly down the hall, passing by numerous patients, who may or may not have noticed me.

We took seats in unmatched chairs around the perimeter of the office. The doc explained that he wanted us to be present for one of his one-on-one client meetings. A young girl came into the office and sat in the chair across from his desk. She had a flat affect and did not acknowledge that we were there. He began to talk. He gestured toward us to indicate that this was not a private session. She stared straight ahead. He opened the meeting by telling the girl he had been on a trip recently and he thought of her while he was there. He bought her a present, in fact. Immediately, questions started popping up in my head. I wondered about the appropriateness of giving a patient a present. Is that ok? *That seems weird*, I thought.

He picked up a wrapped shirt box with light-pink curling ribbon from the floor beside him and stood up to hand it to her over the desk. She took the box. She said nothing. She slowly slid the ribbon off and placed it on her lap. She turned the box over.

She calmly proceeded to slide her finger under the taped edges to release the paper. She tipped the box over and slowly ran her finger between the two meeting edges of the paper. The wrapping fell off onto the floor and she proceeded, almost trancelike, to remove the lid and separate the tissue paper within. A black hooded sweatshirt from The Black Dog lay inside. She did not look up at the doc when he asked if she liked her gift. She did not thank him for it and exhibited no emotion as she released it onto the floor next to her chair. Smoothly, effortlessly, with no hint at the motive behind the action, she gathered the ribbon from her lap, wound it around her neck twice, and began to pull. The psychiatrist continued to sit in his chair as he watched this horrific act. He made little effort to intervene, except to say, "Ok now. That's enough. Stop that."

We continued to watch this girl actively strangle herself a few feet away from us. He ordered us students to stay back and not interfere. The doc finally called a code and headed over to the girl to try and wrestle the ribbon from her grasp as the team barged into the office. Several members did a takedown and pinned her face down into the carpet. The whole time, the doc was saying over and over again to the girl, "We're going to keep you safe. We're here to help you."

The ribbon was finally unwound from her neck. The team escorted her out. I left the unit and drove home. I could not shake my dismay over this unexpected lesson that there were such bad docs out there. It was unsettling that he was still allowed a license to practice medicine. He thought he was God. What made the experience ultimately so awful was the disparity between this psychiatrist and the truly caring and clinically excellent doctors whom I'd had the pleasure of working with up until that point. I had been surrounded by docs emulating exactly how I thought I would hope to practice, so to be confronted by this lack of skill, insight, and care was shocking. I faced a steep learning curve that day.

2

Lessons Learned

As family medicine residents, we rotated through experiences that would ensure we knew the essentials. We spent a lot of time in community care, pediatrics, women's care, and primary care. We also rotated through specialties that were required and others that we chose based on our preferences. We spent time in the hospitals and outpatient clinics. We learned from the residents ahead of us and the attendings ahead of them. We were thrown into some things very quickly, with the expectation being "See one. Do one. Teach one." We also had tremendously kind teachers who took the time to let us practice, fail, learn, and perfect.

As a chief resident, I coordinated with other specialties and managed the schedule of rotations, vacations, educational programming, and teaching. All the while, I was a resident myself. It felt like a three-ring circus some days. But it was worth it. The most memorable lessons came directly from my patients through the process of caring for them.

On one occasion, I was coming in to work my shift in the ED and was taking report from the attending who was finishing up. A new admit had come in just in the last half hour or so. The attending wanted me to keep an eye on her for a couple of hours. Everything looked fine, he assured me. I walked down the hall to introduce myself.

"Why am I here?" she asked as soon as I entered the room.

I was caught off guard, but I answered her. "Oh, you don't remember? You were thrown from your horse."

She looked stunned. "That's strange," she said. "He never does that!"

I let her rest and told her I'd be back to check on her. Half an hour later, I went back to see her. She looked up and smiled. I asked her how she was feeling. She said she was fine. Then she asked why she was there. I hesitated, a little confused. Was she kidding? She didn't look like she was joking around.

I told her again. "You were thrown from your horse."

With a look of utter shock, she replied, "MY horse? He never does that!" She was as rattled as she had been the first time I told her the news. I reassured her she was going to be all right and that we were monitoring her while she recovered.

"Try to rest," I said.

I gave her another fifteen minutes and checked on her again. I was hopeful we would have a different conversation, but no, she asked why she was in the hospital once again.

I walked out of the room, turned the corner, and stopped in the hallway. I wondered how long it would be before she remembered. I waited a moment and then walked right back in.

"Hello!" I said cheerfully as I entered. She looked up and smiled. I was so curious; I started the conversation before she had a chance to talk. "Do you know why you are here?" I asked.

With tears starting to well up in her eyes, she replied, "No. I don't know. Can you tell me? Do you know?"

I suddenly realized that while the neurology of this was fascinating from a medical standpoint, it was frightening to this woman.

I said gently, "You were thrown from your horse." I waited. Her
eyes darted around, processing this information.

"My horse? Really? That's so strange. He never does that," she
replied.

I did my best to comfort her. "That must be quite a surprise
then. I'm sure he didn't mean it."

She was shaking her head. I let her know that some other doctors would be coming in to talk with her and do a scan of her brain
to make sure everything looked all right. She nodded her head and
I wished her good luck as I left the room. Her post-traumatic am-
nesia hadn't resolved by the time I ended of my shift.

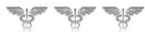

I was moonlighting as the pediatric on-call doc in the ED at the
hospital down the street. A child came into the ED, brought in by
the babysitter. The child was clearly not well: lethargic, not reac-
tive, not acting right. Neither parent was there. I called radiology.

"Can we get some imaging? Head imaging. Can you give me a
couple of plates?" Things started happening very quickly—bang-
bang-bang.

The first plate came back. "Oh my God," I said as I looked at
the image. "This kid has a skull fracture, a facial fracture." My
mind was racing. I tasted bile in my throat. I was angry. What happened to this poor little kid? This kid has been abused—a classic
injury. Who could have done this? Babysitter? Parents? But I
needed to focus. The patient needed me. Care first; figure the rest
out later. At one point, I was on two phones, one on each ear. One
call was with the Level 1 trauma hospital down the road. I was ar-
ranging to transfer the patient.

"Got a kid here," I said. I could feel my heart starting to beat quickly. Their instructions: "Send them down, but only when you can secure an airway. We'll be ready." No one person was any better than anyone else at that point; the goal was to get the airway. We had tried initially, but the kid was alert enough to be resistive. Unless the child was sedated, there was no way to accomplish that.

The other call was to the anesthesiologist. I told him the situation. "Ten minutes," he said. We prepped and waited impatiently. Anesthesiology arrived and dosed the kid. When the child was sedated, they gently placed the trach. The entire team was in there. We lifted the patient, now stable and ready for transfer, onto the gurney, and the paramedics wheeled it out to the bay. The ambulance took two hard rights and passed in front of the hospital, where I was starting to write my notes at the nurses' station. It was late and the city was quiet. I could hear the siren all the way down the long main street to the trauma center. I never heard about what happened to that little kid. When I look back on this, I consider it my first real experience of being a doctor working with a team, under pressure, to care for a patient. The stakes were so high. This was an innocent little kid. This was what I wanted to do. I wanted to be there to help people. This was why we did it. It was a calling.

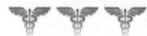

I was working at a community clinic, where I was the doc for a young couple who were expecting their first baby. Over the months, I saw them for care until the big day arrived. Both extended families were at the clinic to support the couple. It was refreshing to see. Everyone was gathered in the room talking with the expectant couple and each other. For a young mom, she was doing really well. As the contractions became closer, the rest of the family headed to the waiting room while the soon-to-be grandmas and the young dad stayed to coach her. The nurses were great with the couple, and we all worked together to explain to them what was happening. I was focused on the mom, coaching her on her timing and waiting to catch the baby. Labor was progressing normally, but quickly. The baby's head began to crown and with it, a fair amount of amniotic fluid and blood spurted out. Immediately, I heard a shriek. I had to raise myself off the exam stool and saw the young dad looking on in horror. He was inconsolable and began to hyper-ventilate. I was not sure what was going on with him, but I did know that I was still in the middle of the delivery and did not want him distressing the young mom. I told one of the nurses to get him out of the room. Flanking him, a nurse and his mother helped him into the hallway. I heard the commotion behind me. All the while, the young mom labored and soon delivered a beautiful, healthy baby. With no repair needed, I concentrated on the one- and five-minute Apgars. Within minutes, one of the nurses led the pale and clammy young dad back into the room. I held up the baby and congratulated him. He started to sob and had to sit down. After a minute, he was able to choke out, "I thought you pulled his head off." It took him about half an hour to calm down.

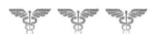

I was doing a rotation in the ICU and was scheduled to be on call every three days. It certainly felt like my "days on" came quicker than that; it was physically and mentally exhausting work, and I was the new guy. I dragged myself in and was met by a nurse who informed me of my first task of the day: There had been a death on the unit, and I needed to call it. The panicked expression on my face gave me away—I had no idea what to do. It was July and I was a first-year resident. I had only been doing this for a month. I fol-lowed her down the hall. She was patient and guided me through the process: Feel for a pulse at the carotid artery. Check the eyes for pupillary reaction. Listen for spontaneous breathing. Write your name on the bottom of this form and pronounce the death. It seemed like something so significant should have involved more than that. I took a deep breath and, with a flourish, I proclaimed, "You're dead," over the body. I turned to the nurse for approval. She gave me a blank stare and said flatly, "Great." She then rolled her eyes, marked the time, and left the room. I realized immediately from her reaction that "pronounce" meant something very different than "announce." I still had a lot left to learn.

3

Relationships Made

I t is the relationship with the family, and with the patient, that is most important. Sometimes care involves exchanges as intimate as one would have with family. People share with you their deepest feelings, their fears. You follow people through life, through good times and bad. You are witness to it; sometimes you are part of it. These are experiences that will keep coming back to you.

I always had an open-door policy for my staff. I spent more time with my patients when they needed it; I saw them off-hours if it was easier for them. I did make home visits when people couldn't easily get to me. You can't really know people fully until you've been invited into their homes. I went to games even though it wasn't my kid playing. I went to the wakes. It's what you do. It isn't easy, but that's your role. Birth to death. We aim to foster a community.

These days, many primary care providers (PCPs) are willing to treat their patients through telemedicine. This works if they already have a relationship with the patient. As a PCP, you are "on" 24-7. I've talked with many PCPs around the country who are burnt out. The system has broken them. They've ended up in a place where they treat the ailment and they treat it well, but they have neither the time nor the bandwidth to treat the patient. Even during my time as a doc, independent private practices were, by far, better able than large hospital systems at fostering patient relationships. Docs in these practices liked the fact that they could give their patients more time. They would have loved to stay independent, but it's getting harder and harder, they would tell me. The administrative work, the billing, the coding. They worried that the big hospitals would get even bigger and independent practices would become obsolete. They would try and link up with the community hospitals for support, but these didn't have a lot of resources either. I often brought up the idea of bridging the gap by affiliating with a larger hospital system to use their resources and get incentives to have your patients use the services. That way, a doc could still stay independent but have support if they needed it.

I've talked with many docs, good and bad. One said, "I really don't do much. I do an exam and if someone needs anything else, I start a referral. The medical assistants do the rest." My point is, how do we call that care? It's expensive. It's not comprehensive. It's not patient centered. Care is often incentive driven and strictly time managed.

Urgent care centers have entered the scene. A provider working there might say, "This is so easy. Rather than having to know everything about a patient, I have just one thing to treat." The problem is, this is someone's life. There's no continuity of care. You need to know your patients' stories. You need to know what the priorities are. You need to know who the people in their lives are. You need to treat the whole person.

Finding a good PCP is like dating. You don't know what you've got when you first start seeing a person, but after a few dates, you

have a better sense of whether the relationship is going some-
where. Sometimes, it's quick and you know right away—"this is a
doc who will listen, who will partner with me, and who I feel comfortable with—this is exactly what I need."

I've had patients with me for as long as I've been practicing as
an independent physician. Having good, mutual communication
and respect is essential. A patient will come in and they want
something; maybe they are in pain and they are asking for a pain-
killer. Physicians need to think about the whole picture: What is
going on? What do we need to investigate further? If someone has
respect and trust in you, they are going to listen; they are going to
allow the time to walk down that path. If there is pushback or if
someone is demanding, it sets off your radar. You have to match
the problem with the solution. Good medicine isn't based on knee-
jerk reactions or poor planning.

For my patients, I would open the door and ask, "How are you
doing? What can I do for you?" Then I would listen. If I needed
more information, I might ask some pointed questions, but usually,
just letting the patient talk would eventually provide the information I was looking for. I wanted patients to feel they were getting
better. I gave them time to be heard. You can't do good medicine in
a hurry; if you do, not only does the patient not get the care they
need, your relationship with the patient also suffers. Rather than
"You've got fifteen minutes" (what can you do in such a short
time?), if you give patients time to build a relationship with you,
they open up.

I tried to get my patients in as quickly as possible if they had
an urgent concern. Stay late; put them at the end of the day; see
them over lunch; fit them in to a cancellation; or somehow find a
few minutes during the day.

I tried to meet people where they were at. For example,
sometimes as a kid, you have to get a vaccine. They are not fun but
it's something you need to do to stay healthy. It's a tough lesson for

a kid, but at some point, after all the rationalizing, you just have to tell them, gently, to get over themselves. And that's when I belt out the theme from *Frozen* in the hallway. Seeing your doc act like a fool singing "Let it go! Let it go!" usually works wonders for breaking down barriers. The staff liked it too.

Be humble. Don't take yourself too seriously. Do what works.

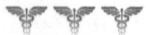

I happened to have this young pregnant girl on my caseload one day. She was probably about fifteen years old. She was starting care at the clinic where I was working. I did an exam and found everything was going well, progress consistent with dates. We went over the plan for the next few weeks. Her biggest ask was to know the gender of the baby. I disappointed her by letting her know that protocol didn't allow us to do an ultrasound unless there was a medical need for it. Plus, an unborn baby's sex can be one of the last few unknowns left in modern life—surely she'd want to be surprised? I told her I would see her back in a month.

A month later, I was in the clinic again. I looked over my patient's record before entering the room and read she had experienced some spotting a week prior, necessitating an ultrasound.

After a routine exam that showed nothing out of the ordinary, I said "Great! You are doing well, and now you know what sex the baby is!"

She grinned. "Yup!"

A moment passed.

"Well?" I said excitedly. "What is it?"

She was still grinning at me. "I'm not telling you! You didn't want to know."

I was a little surprised. Sassy little kid. But I laughed at her mettle. Each visit, no news for me. I guessed I'd have to wait and see.

The call came in that she was in labor. I met her at the hospital.

The attending physician let me know he was just leaving his house, about an hour's drive away. Labor was progressing quickly, so the nurses prepped and I readied for what looked likely to be a solo delivery—my first. Questions raced through my mind. *Is this going to be a normal delivery? Is the mom going to be strong enough to labor well and listen to the coaching? Will we have to worry about the baby's breathing after they're born? What about the cord?*

Whatever worries I had, it was go time. After the head crowned, I delivered the head, then the right shoulder, left shoulder, and supported the weight of the baby as the legs emerged. The baby was out, but there was more to do: hold the slippery baby up and show the mom her little one, then suction, then wipe down the baby, then Apgar scores, and then lay the baby on the mom. It was a stressful few minutes. I wanted to get everything right. I stopped to take in the situation: Mom and baby doing well. Nurses working as a team to attend to Mom and baby. I had caught my first baby solo and it all went fine. I let out a breath. The mom looked to me and smiled.

"Now you know, Dr. Brown!"

"Sorry?" It took me a moment to register the comment.

"Now you know the sex of the baby!"

Stunned, I realized that with everything going on, I hadn't looked.

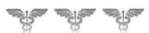

A woman came into the office to confirm a pregnancy. A positive test came back, and she was overjoyed. It was her eighth pregnancy. While she had carried babies through pregnancy successfully, she had also experienced multiple spontaneous miscarriages. She fell into the high-risk category, both because of her age and her multiple pregnancies. We discussed transfer to the obstetrics (OB) service; however, we felt she could be treated appropriately through our practice, and she indicated a preference to stay with us. I read over everything I could on high-risk pregnancies and treatment. I followed this woman through her pregnancy. No issues. Proceeding well.

It was a few weeks later. The early stages of labor began, and the woman came to the hospital. We placed a monitor and watched the baby's heart rate. The line dipped, but recovered back to baseline, dipped again and recovered once more. From the research I had done, I felt we could keep the woman on service, and the chief confirmed my research and my decision. The family practice residents and the OB who came for a consult argued back and forth over the baby's heart-rate monitoring. The OB thought she should have a C-section, but there was no reason for it. The spikes were a good sign: They indicated that the baby was able to recover from the stress of the contractions. Between all of the docs and nursing staff, the room was full and loud. A small voice emerged from the back of the room amid all the arguing. Everyone stopped and turned toward the woman. We heard my patient say, "But, Dr. Brown, Dr. Brown, you're my doctor." The team regrouped. We made the decision to proceed as planned. Delivery was uneventful. Baby was perfect. Mom was joyful.

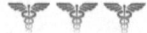

A family I knew brought their newborn in for a visit. Another doc had seen the baby; the mom was concerned about a lump she had found while bathing the baby. The doc thought it was unremarkable, but the mom still seemed worried. I met up with her as she was leaving the exam room.

"Dr. Brown, I found this lump."

I asked if I could examine the baby. I palpated a spongy mass in the baby's abdomen that should not have been there. After some quick research to confirm my dire suspicions, I discussed the findings with the mom and was blunt: This baby needed medical imaging immediately. I suspected a mesoblastic nephroma—a tumor, usually found in newborns, that grows rapidly. The baby was scheduled for an MRI that day at Children's Hospital, followed by a biopsy the next day. The cancer was diagnosed within hours, and the baby was scheduled for surgery a day later. I was in contact with the family, who was obviously in a state of shock. The baby made it through surgery without complications, and then the long, slow recovery began. Radiation, chemo, follow-up visits, overnight stays in the hospital for the baby and the mom, the emotional toll of watching your baby have to be sedated for treatments five days a week for months, not to mention other challenges—suddenly living on one paycheck, still caring for another child, financial burdens from health care and leave, struggles to maintain normal relationships with family and friends, and the constant worry: What if they didn't get it all?

There are always families whose struggles touch your heart, and this one in particular remained at the forefront of my mind. Over the years, I traveled the path with them. I received reports from her oncologist. I fundraised for them. I continued to be her doc. She nicknamed me "Uncle Brown." I received a text the other day from the mom: "Still cancer-free. Kidney looks great." More than a decade later, I still feel honored to have been her doc and cherish the relationship that the family and I still share.

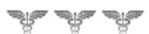

I had another patient who traveled extensively. He received grants to travel to international locations in need of aid and would stay on for months to support various agencies. Whenever he was preparing for a trip, he would give me a call and ask if we had any expired medications or medical supplies that we would feel comfortable donating. The relief agencies would take whatever we were willing to part with. I would always say "Yes, of course."

During one of his overseas visits, he unfortunately was involved in a car accident. The taxi he was in skidded off a rural dirt road into an embankment. He sustained a laceration on his forehead that required suturing. The medics stitched him up and gave him instructions to keep the dressing on and keep it dry and clean. He did what he could while out of the country and came in to see me when he returned home. I heard about the incident just before he arrived at the office and was curious to see how rough the injury was. It wasn't bad. I truly thought it would look worse. The wound was healing; it wasn't infected. This was a welcome surprise, given that my patient was in the middle of nowhere and the sutures the medics had used were so thick they looked like they came off a skein of blue yarn. I can say that despite the guy's strength of spirit for his calling, medical procedures were not easy for him to endure. We took it slowly. The session, including suture removal, debriding, irrigation, and rebandaging, took about two hours. He walked out of the office with a ten-day prescription for antibiotics and instructions to call me if the wound started to look red or irritated. I had faith he was healing well and could take it on his own from there.

This same patient happened to live nearby our small town. The next time I saw him was when I made an emergency house call. He had fallen in his yard and turned his ankle. He couldn't walk. He sent his daughter out on her bike with explicit directions to "Go get Doc Brown!" I obviously didn't hesitate, jumping in the car and bringing his daughter and her bike back to their house. He ended up being fine. It was just a sprain. I bandaged him and told him to follow up in the office the next day. I was pleased he trusted me enough to be his first line of defense. I also think about how the instructions he gave his daughter made it sound like we lived out on the prairie a century ago.

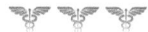

A retired army guy decided he wanted to fulfill a lifelong dream and parachute out of a plane for his birthday. He was turning eighty-three. He and his wife, also my patient, came in for his appointment. He needed my permission to complete the tandem jump. He had a coy smile and appeared somewhat giddy. His wife, who was looking on skeptically, was clearly not on board with this idea and was hoping that I'd back the decision to ground him. She began her argument: "He wants to jump out of a plane. That's crazy, right? Talk to him, Doc." She was nearly hyperventilating. She turned toward her husband, who was sitting on the exam table, relaxed and looking somewhat disinterested in the conversation.

"You could die!" she blurted out.

A man of few words, the husband replied dryly, "Yes, we went over that."

"Seriously, you could die!" she exclaimed. She looked scared.

"I could die tomorrow." He looked up and shrugged his shoulders.

They both turned to me.

She expected that I would, of course, say no. You could tell that they'd argued this many times before. I turned to the husband and asked him, "Are you okay with the worst-case scenario? Are you okay with dying during this jump?"

He didn't hesitate: "Yep. I'm old."

"Okay," I said to him. "You could die, but you are healthy enough to go through with this."

The wife had now lost the one person who might have been able to put an end to this nonsense. She left the room in a quiet boil, with a look of absolute disappointment.

I heard later that he had done the jump successfully. Read it in the local paper. Made the front page.

After years of seeing this same couple as patients, the wife began to decline. Her family took great care of her. She would come to the office in a new minivan, upgraded with a lift for her wheelchair. When she wasn't feeling strong enough to come in, I went to her house to see her. The husband called the office one day. When I got back to him, he let me know that he and the family were making arrangements for his wife to be transferred to a hospice facility. She was on my mind all night. The next morning I called to ask if I could do a home visit prior to her transfer. I knew it would probably be the last time I saw her. I just wanted to say goodbye. The husband, stoic and quiet, greeted me at the door. I followed him down the hall to her room. I looked at the wife. She was peaceful. She probably didn't know I was there. I turned to the husband.

"Do you mind if I kiss her goodbye?"

He stepped back to let me pass. I kissed her on the cheek, then quickly left the room. I was sad. Saying a final goodbye to a patient is never easy. Her extended family had gathered in the kitchen and were having a frank discussion about end-of-life care. They stopped talking as I entered the room. I introduced myself and gave my condolences to the group. I left them to their planning. She passed a few days later.

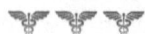

I had just joined a tiny, stand-alone family practice with a couple of docs and a nurse practitioner. I was a month or two out of residency at a major teaching hospital. My new home was a community hospital in an old manufacturing town. I was on call for the first time and I received a page from the ED.

"You've got a kiddo!"

I hopped in the car and received the report from one of the nurses on duty. A three-month-old baby, a patient of the practice, had been brought in with a high fever. This little one needed a lumbar puncture (LP) and time was of the essence. I directed the staff as best I could to set up for treatment ahead of my arrival and asked them to have at the ready one pediatric LP kit and a seasoned nurse who could hold a baby securely. The area at the lumbar spine had to remain sterile. There could be no movement during the procedure. This LP procedure would require a bit more finesse than usual. While the placement of a needle in an adult is usually around the level of the fourth or fifth lumbar vertebra, in a three-month-old, the spine is so tiny that it is hard to tell which vertebra you are at. And whereas the spinal canal where the cerebrospinal fluid is drawn from is about an inch wide in an adult, it is only a few millimeters in a baby this young.

I trucked down the road quickly; there was no traffic given the late hour. I parked close to where I thought the ED entrance was. Having never been there before, I did not know exactly where to go, nor did anyone know who I was when I walked in. When I arrived, they looked at me like my presence was some kind of joke. I thought it was because I was a very young-looking doc, fresh out of training. (My nickname was Doogie in medical school.) I met the parents and explained the procedure. I was then directed to a room where a calm but determined-looking nurse stood over a small plastic crib where a tiny baby girl was asleep, ready to be prepped for the procedure. The tray next to the crib was laid out with the instruments I had requested. In my experience this procedure generally worked better with fewer people in the room, so having only one other person with me was ideal. The nurse did a fantastic job positioning the baby properly and holding her firmly in place. From the needle insertion to the draw to the removal, the whole procedure took about six or seven minutes. I sent the sample out stat and then went out to the waiting area to talk with the parents, who were understandably concerned. I reassured them that all went well and that I would follow up with the results, which should be back within the hour. The labs came back positive for a bacterial infection. I spoke with the parents about next steps—overnight stay with some intravenous (IV) antibiotics and monitoring through the night. They expressed their appreciation and agreed to follow up in the office once the baby was discharged. I wrote up my notes and headed home.

The following day, I reached out to my colleague to give sign-out. There were no hospitalists at this hospital at the time, so community docs went in and did patient rounds. My colleague looked at me a bit askance, with an expression not unsimilar to the look I got walking into the ED the night before.

"Why would you do an LP on a three-month-old?" she gasped.

"She needed one." I replied.

"I would have sent her to the Children's Hospital. No one does that at a community hospital," she retorted.

Ah. That's why everyone had looked at me funny.

Yet, I felt a bit confused. Why would I send the family an hour down the road, when I was perfectly capable of doing a procedure five minutes from their house?

The baby rebounded well and came into the office not just for a follow-up, but for the next twenty-four years. She continued to be a patient at the practice. I was able to be her doc for the first twelve or so years of her life, until she divulged that she would be more comfortable seeing a "girl doctor" at our practice. The parents remained my patients until I retired. At each visit, they talked about that night in the ED.

4

Clinical Pearls: What to Do and What Not to Do

D ocs are human. They are going to make mistakes. Not necessarily medical mistakes, but not having your heart and your head in the game can cause some significant damage. Some are hard to forget. I recall one woman on the maternity unit when I was shadowing rounds as a student. The attending led a group of us into the room and he proceeded to ask her how her baby was doing. She suddenly broke down and choked out that her baby had died. The attending quickly apologized and then hightailed it out of the room. It was a primer in what not to do. Why hadn't he checked the chart before he went in? Or asked the nurses how the patient was doing? Or gotten report from the doc on call? These were critically important steps to avoid making a patient feel worse.

I've had many students over the course of my medical career. There are lessons you can teach—suturing, diabetes management, hypertension education and treatment—but other knowledge is harder to impart. You have to have someone show you. You have to observe someone who believes in the principles of patient-centered care, active listening, the importance of collaboration. You have to start with someone who is willing to practice in this way. We took the Hippocratic oath at graduation from medical school, but day to day I was basing my approach to treatment on my own personal ethics. One shouldn't need a poem to tell you how to act; the guiding principles of medicine are hopefully in you already and can be fostered by a mentor. You are bound to them. You hold yourself accountable. It transcends all and applies to everything you do.

I tried to be compassionate and collaborative, and strived to provide health education to my patients so they could make their own meaningful choices. Fostering this mindset in students is hard. Really hard. But I always liked teaching. Give me a brand-new medical student and I'm happy. Everyone needs a good foundation, a good start. I hope I was able to pass those lessons on to my students through my actions.

One of my strongest mentors was a stellar nurse practitioner, a kind soul, who set the tone for the office. She called to check on her patients, not just for medical follow-up, but simply to see how life events they had discussed in recent visits had gone. She saw patients for as long as they needed in their sessions. Her other patients waited patiently if she was running late because they knew they would be afforded the same privilege of time and active listening. As a medical provider, you do this because it's the right thing to do. I understood that I was going to be running late at the office—a lot. I was seeing patients for as long as they needed, seeing patients after hours, calling them back, making sure their questions were answered and their fears were allayed.

It is callous system that requires you to put a name and a five-digit code on a visit with a patient—as though that's all a person is worth. You could be talking about life-changing events. In the hospitals, it is even worse. You choose a billing code for the highest amount you can charge. How can you hold yourself to a higher benchmark when you are tired, overworked, overwhelmed?

First, you have to like what you are doing. You have to like your patients. People were asking for help, and I was giving them the help they needed. In the practice, I also was one of the only ones doing certain procedures: removing ingrown toenails, lancing sebaceous cysts, injecting cortisone into joints. I felt a heightened level of responsibility, but I loved doing them—they were fun. I also enjoyed my interactions with kids. I acted goofy and tried to make the appointment as fun as possible. I didn't want them to be scared to come in. I wanted them to feel it was a safe space.

One of my most impactful cases began when a gentleman was in need of a new PCP. His wife was a patient in our practice, and she asked if I might be available to take him on. I was happy to add him to my panel. On his first visit, he arrived in a power chair accompanied by his wife. She was his voice; he was essentially nonverbal. His diagnosis was amyotrophic lateral sclerosis (ALS). They traveled; they went hiking; she would put him in their wheelchair van and off they went. Her attitude was "Come on. Let's go. That's why we got this thing."

She was damned if he was going to stay home and just waste away. It got to the point that I would call the house before a home visit because they were on the road so much. They would apologize if a trip coincided with a visit, but I just cheered them on. That was important. No one else wanted to take him on as a patient; docs didn't feel comfortable about the disease process. The ironic thing was that he was relatively healthy, with no need for chronic disease management. The main thing he needed was good care and help with planning for the inevitable. We addressed pain management, community resource ideas, care partner support, home modifications, setting up services for the future, and ideas to make his quality of life better. No one could cure his ALS, but we could make his life as good as it could be. It was easy in one sense—just be responsive and supportive of their choices. Some visits were no big deal—simply check in and make sure things were going all right. Other visits were fraught with anxiety or frustration. His wife needed me to do something to get the ball rolling: to authorize a service, to sign a form. I always reassured her that I would help and that she could take that off her list. Her husband still had facial expressions. He still laughed. I loved when something I said made him utter a hearty "Heh-heh."

I was in awe of their relationship. ALS is the kind of thing that can ruin a marriage. I was humbled by his situation and by the way his wife was caring for him. What if that were me? What if my family were in that situation? She wanted him to live and to have the best quality of life that he could, even under these circumstances.

When it made sense to start doing home care, there was almost always someone at the house. As he became more disabled, his wife found herself having to search for more and more support for him, even as the options slowly waned. The disease progressed, and his wife ended up doing anything he needed. She researched and found the best gel pad for his bed that money could buy; she learned the best way to massage him to help alleviate the pain from the crushing muscle contractions he experienced; they engaged a care team to come into their home. I ordered whatever he needed. He had physical therapy at home, but it wasn't a good fit for the family. He had speech therapy. They tried a speech-generating device, but that was quickly abandoned. His wife kept in touch with the ALS Association. She modified the house with a ramp, an accessible bedroom, and shower. She jumped through the hoops to get him set up with social security disability insurance and Medicare.

As time went on, his condition continued to deteriorate. I got a call one day from the hospice nurse: "He hasn't slept for three days. He's in pain." I signed the orders to increase the morphine in the drip. Over the course of forty-eight hours, I received numerous calls from the hospice nurse for more increases in the dose. The pain just wasn't under control, and he still hadn't slept. By the end of the second day, he was on a gram of morphine around the clock, and it still wasn't helping him. A few hours later, after I had finished up with my other patients, I went to the house. His wife was sad when she opened the door, clearly concerned that this was the beginning of the end. Before I even stepped over the threshold in the house, I could see him, his eyes wide open, looking toward me. He watched me intently as I walked down the hall. I had never seen him like that before. There was obviously something wrong. He looked scared. He was pleading for help. I spoke with him, hoping to calm him down. I started to panic and could feel my heart racing as I saw how much pain he was in.

Steadying my voice as much as I could, I said, "It's okay, it's okay. I'm going to help. We're going to get you something for the pain."

I quickly started a brief exam but went easy because I didn't want to add to the pain. His abdomen was distended. I looked down at the line from the catheter. I looked at the bag. Empty. I asked when he voided last. The wife reported it had been days, but that the nurse said that was to be expected.

"Anybody think to change the catheter?" I said, more to myself.

The wife stopped moving and looked at me with disbelief. "Oh my God. Could that be it?"

I thought, *That's it. I'm taking control.*

I explained the situation to him. "I think your catheter is blocked. I'm going to change it."

He looked at me and watched as I turned to march toward the kitchen where the stores of medical supplies were kept. I was so angry. No one should ever be in this much pain. I rummaged through the boxes and found a catheter, washed my hands in the kitchen sink, and hurried back to the bedroom.

I placed the equipment on a small table his wife had set up. She stood next to him, her arm draped over his shoulders, watching intently. He looked on as I slowly removed the old catheter. I flushed the new catheter with about 10 ccs of saline and slid it into place. The urine started flowing immediately. I looked up at him. He looked back at me and sighed. He closed his eyes and within seconds, he was asleep. I sighed. "Sleep well," I said in my head.

His wife, meanwhile, had stomped down the hall, yelling obscenities. Intermittently, I could hear her repeat, "How could they do that?"

I picked up the trash and threw the old catheter into the red medical waste bag in his room. He was still sleeping soundly. I left his room and headed into the kitchen. His wife was standing, arms folded, leaning against the counter. She informed me that she had just fired the hospice agency—on the spot. I wasn't surprised. She was an incredible advocate for her husband and only wanted the best for him.

I left the family and headed home. The ride home was a blur. It was one of the most horrific things I'd seen a person go through. Imagine having to die that way? You can't tell anyone. You can't scream.

Within a few months, he passed away. His wife called me when he died, and I went to the house. His passing was expected, but it was not easy, especially because he had kids. I sat next to him on the couch. I didn't remove the IVs. I didn't take out his catheter. I didn't remove any tubes. We just sat with him, each kid taking a turn, his wife sitting next to him. They talked to him, his wife talked to their children. We tried to make the youngest child, in his late teens, as comfortable as possible with the situation. The funeral director arrived, and my patient left his house for the last time. I spent a little more time talking with the family and then went home.

I went to the wake. It's what you do. His wife was gracious and thankful. She had gone through a long mourning period as her husband declined. She was incredibly strong. I took the kids on as patients when they asked—all of them. I did what I could to support them in any way I could. They stayed, in a safe space, for a time and then slowly left the practice.

Clinical pearl: Know your patient, listen to your patient. He could not talk but his face said everything. Trust your gut and, in the words attributed to Dr. Theodore Woodward, "When you hear hoof beats, think horses, not zebras."

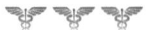

A long-standing patient came in for a visit. We had maintained a good relationship over many years. During the exam, he noted that he was a little worried about his memory. Nothing big, but things like forgetting where he left the car keys or his glasses. I completed a series of cognitive screenings on him. Nothing of concern showed up. I would have expected a dip in performance on any of these tests if there were something to be worried about. I listened as he described his day-to-day functioning. No issues. I could have sent him to neurology, but I was not impressed. He took me at my word.

On a subsequent visit, my patient's wife came in with him. She wasn't convinced of my findings. I was comfortable ordering some bloodwork. I started to talk with the husband, asking him about any concerns about cognitive functioning and explaining normal aging.

We were in the middle of talking when the wife interjected, "Oh, don't bother telling him anything. He's just going to forget it in five minutes." It caught me off guard. I thought it was just so sad, so cruel. I was dumbfounded. I looked at her. And then back at him. He shrugged a bit and looked embarrassed. Even if there were cognitive changes going on, he had enough understanding to know that he was being belittled. I sighed. I thought to myself,

What would he say if he could? If he could find the words to accurately express how he was feeling at that moment?

Did his wife love him? Did she think the person he had been was gone? Was he just inconsequential to her? Now you have a pattern—now he doesn't get the opportunity to talk at all. It cuts deep. It was hard to know what happened between them outside of the office. Would what I say make it worse? I felt bad for him. Neither he nor I said anything. I didn't feel it was my place to say anything. I didn't want to make their relationship tougher. It was always that whatever the wife says, goes. And it was their last visit with me. They were going to get care at another office. He had to leave and be cared for by this woman. The encounter was very unpleasant.

Another of my patients came in for a visit and she was clearly more impaired than before. She didn't know why she was there. She was brought into the visit by her husband and their daughter. Sweetest guy. I tried to make her yearly physical a pleasant interaction. She was cooperative but clearly annoyed and kept uttering, "I just don't know why I'm here."

The husband was calm, patient, and very attentive despite the many times she repeated this. No anger, no annoyance. Just answered her question over and over again and reassured her. "You are here to see Dr. Brown for your checkup."

After the visit, I walked them out and had a chance to talk with the husband as we were a few feet behind the patient and their daughter.

"Wow. You are amazing. How do you do it? She asked the same question over and over again and you just answered it without getting frustrated. Don't you get tired of that?"

He said matter-of-factly, "No. I love her. I respond like it is the first time she is asking it, because to her, it is."

Clinical pearl: Both this and the previous circumstance made me appreciate more than ever the importance of preserving dignity and showing kindness, to any fellow human being, especially someone you love.

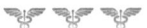

One of the best teachers I learned from was a boisterous hospice doc with a thick brogue and a propensity to call people out for what he deemed shallow responses. The thing that drew him to me was that he earnestly cared for people. He brought people together. He introduced me to the concept of the family meeting. This was a method of helping people cope with the impending death of a loved one. He would meet people in their homes. He would go to hospice facilities. It wasn't orchestrated or scheduled; he would just gather people who were there visiting. Everyone was at a different point. Some were stoic; they weren't ready yet. Some were unabashedly crying over a loss, whether it was the one they were anticipating or a past loss. Some folks would apologize for thinking of other losses in that moment, but he would encourage them to speak. They hadn't grieved fully; they hadn't started the healing process. This was a perfect opportunity to do it. Random family members, friends were gathered. He brought people together. "Tell me about your person." If you glossed over the issue or decided you didn't want to reveal your true feelings, he would encourage you; he would challenge you: "Bullshit!"

People would open up. Doing this allowed them the chance to come to terms with loss and put things into true perspective: "Other people are grieving. Maybe my problems are not so bad. I know what I need to do now." It was this doctor's life's love. It was touching. He healed people who didn't even realize they were hurting. It happened in the moment; there was no planning for something like this. The expertise came from knowing when the time was right to gather everyone. There was no requirement to talk; people could pass. But he knew when people were hurting, and he would draw them out. It drained everyone there, physically and emotionally, but people expressed relief, gratitude, and peace after the meeting. It wasn't for the person who was dying; it was for the family. It was fluid; it changed as the family needed it to.

I ran a family meeting whenever I could because I knew how helpful it was for my patients. It was medicine. I didn't bill for a family meeting. As the facilitator, I invited people to join. Whether the dying family member was present, as they were at some meetings, or not, the family could still work through the issues. Sometimes people had conflicting ideas, but each person had a chance to speak. In general, these meetings went well. The facilitator stepped in to make connections between the many thoughts that were brought up to help everyone process the information. There was tension. So many people had thoughts, sometimes it took a while before they were comfortable sharing. Folks were asked to sit in a large circle and went in order, sharing their thoughts; but when it came around to the next round, people often jumped in to reply to something that was said. It was the facilitator's job to keep the flow going smoothly and keep the group discussion to one person at a time.

Facilitators also responded to nonverbal language or asked folks to comment on someone's thoughts, especially if it looked like they might not agree. The facilitator read the room the entire time. "Bullshit"—they called people out to find out the root of the issue, not just skim the surface: "That's what so-and-so should have done twenty years ago." I never had a family meeting devolve into a brawl, but there were some heated discussions. In the end, the feedback was always positive. The meeting served the purpose of bringing to light people's thoughts and emotions so they could process the situation at hand.

Clinical pearl: Do the family meeting. Expect the unexpected. Things will happen. It's emotional, but it's cathartic.

5

Things That Make You Go Hmmm . . .

I was fifty-two years old. Life was busy. It was hard to balance everything, but it was a conscious decision to take it all on. I had been training for a half marathon. My wife and I were making time as a couple for a date night every week and squeezing in a vacation—just us. We enjoyed each other's company and made each other laugh. And I wanted to always be there for the kids. I loved being involved in the things they did. I coached the kids in golf (this was like herding cats), volunteered with them, took them on vacation or to the beach, hurried home to attend parent nights, dressed up and walked around the neighborhood with them on Halloween, taught them how to drive, and moved them into their college dorms. I attended their sporting events, concerts, and plays. We spent game-day Sundays together listening to music, hanging out in our comfy clothes, playing board games, and eating snacks all afternoon. My kids always said, "Daddy's silly." I tried to be protective of the kids' privacy, but it was hard not to talk about them to anyone. They're great kids.

We had the luxury of being able to take the kids to work while I went in on the weekends to catch up on things. We made it fun. It meant sitting at the front desk, playing with stickers and markers, asking us through the sliding window if we needed a "doctor point," punching in numbers on the ancient adding machine, running down the halls and ducking into exam rooms, and then visiting residents at the nursing home.

But I could feel something was up. Professionally, no one saw me on enough of a regular basis to notice anything different in my interactions with the docs or my performance. My role as the CMO of a health-care system had me traveling to our service area across the country. Florida to Louisiana to Texas to Boston. At the practice, we were all busy, and few could weigh in on any changes I might have been showing.

I asked my peers if I was speaking any differently. They suggested I might just be tired, which I was. I was very tired, but that comes with the territory. There was always a pull on both sides. If I was at work, I wanted to be home; if I was home, I felt like I should be at work. If anything good came of COVID, it was that I stopped traveling and I attended meetings virtually from home. I lightened my direct patient hours and was happy to have the extra time to breathe and see my family more.

It was a Friday. I was at my last appointment of the day, a routine physical on a patient I had been seeing for years. I grabbed my stethoscope to recheck his blood pressure. I hesitated. Something wasn't right. I couldn't figure out how to use my stethoscope. I stared at the bell, then looked over at the ear tips. I shifted it around in my hands, stretched it out, and felt each end, until it all started to come back to me. The confusion only lasted a few seconds, but it seemed much longer. My patient noticed the momentary delay.

"Senior moment, Doc?"

I laughed and made some self-deprecating joke. I continued the exam and finished without incident.

But the whole time I was thinking, *That was weird.*

As I drove home that evening, I was truly rattled. It was hard to shake the feeling of dread. So many thoughts were coming, one after the other.

I had remembered asking people, "Do you ever hear me having trouble finding words?"

"No, you're good," they all had said.

I told myself maybe it was nothing significant, just little things that were different here and there. Maybe I don't need to be concerned. But I always came back to thinking, *No, things just aren't right.*

The possible scenarios playing out in my head were unnerving. It boiled down to a couple of thoughts: *I know I have to go to see someone, but I'm afraid of what I'm going to find out.* And then, *Whatever is going on, I don't want to be a burden.*

The neurologist I saw was a colleague. He did me the great favor of getting me in the next business day. He ran through the neuro exam; it felt unremarkable to me.

Again, my thoughts were racing: *What did I agree to? I'm fine. This was a mistake. This is a waste of time. I'm reading into things.*

The nurse practitioner (NP) came in next to administer some baseline testing. She was smart and sassy with a lightning-quick sense of humor.

Mini-mental? I thought. *Sure. Easy. I've given these a bunch of times before. No big deal. Sure. I'll do your test.*

My thoughts went back to my patient: *Apple. Penny. Car.* I let my imagination consider the most surreal possibilities, but just for a moment.

Next came the Montreal Cognitive Assessment, or the MoCA, a cognitive screening that included some drawing tasks.

Ok, I'm not good at drawing. My clock looks messy; my cube looks misshapen.

Another section of that screening, this time part B of the Trail

Making Test. *I'm really not understanding what this is.* Then some math. "Subtract 7 from 100." *Hmmm. Tough.*

On the five-word recall I got three. With hints. (I asked Maureen later what the words were in the car and practiced the whole way home.) I didn't know exactly what was happening with me, but I knew enough to understand that this was not going well, and I thought, *That's it. I'm done. I'm no longer a practicing doc.* I decided right there, right then, in that room.

I took time off. Weeks. It was unprecedented for me. There were more tests to be done, appointments to keep, conversations to have.

I wasn't prepared for any diagnosis, but I tried to convince myself "until it is, it isn't." It didn't work. My brain was going to bad places. I thought, *I'm done. I've got what Robin Williams had.* Then I thought, *No, I've got what my patient had. I have ALS.*

We didn't want to upset our kids. On the way home from appointments, we would pull over into the parking lot of the trailhead near our house. We sobbed on each other's shoulders. We placed our bets on differential diagnoses: frontotemporal dementia (FTD), ALS, Lewy body dementia. As crazy as it sounds, we hoped for a brain tumor. Something you could basically just have scooped out and then go on with your life.

More testing followed: bloodwork, MRI, EEG. I politely declined the lumbar puncture and the neuropsych exam. We got results in spurts in the coming weeks, often while we were in that same parking lot. It wasn't a prion disease; it wasn't tick-borne; it wasn't hypothyroid disease. And it wasn't a tumor. More testing: an FDG-PET scan.

Imagine this. You are about to have a brain scan. There's an IV pushing radioactive glucose through your veins. But that takes time to circulate, so you are put in a small closet, the lights are turned off, and you are told to not use your phone and try to relax and not think of anything. As the nurse closes the door just so, leaving it slightly ajar, she says firmly, "Don't fall asleep."

And that's where I found myself. In a small, dark room. There was a cabinet in front of me that I could just make out in the sliver of light coming through from the hallway. I concentrated on the lines of that cabinet, willing myself not to drift asleep; I didn't want to have to do this again. Time was hard to assess, but it seemed like I was sitting there for about half an hour. When the wait was over, a nurse led me down the hall and over a threshold into the attached modular building that contained the imaging device. Given the wait and the buildup, I figured it would be a long ordeal, but just two minutes and some beeping later, I was on my way out to the waiting room. I was ready to get out of there. The scan had been presented to us as the final test to determine my diagnosis, and the prospect of not needing any more testing made me happy. Plus, we would also have some answers.

Six days later, we had a telemedicine visit with the NP. She gave us the news.

"It's Alzheimer's."

I told her we had read the results already. She asked how I was doing.

I told her I was relieved. "It's *only* Alzheimer's."

Being naive, I thought, *It's not ALS. We can deal with that.* I told the NP and reassured my wife that I'd had patients who lived a long time with Alzheimer's before they had any issues. Looking back now, I feel like I angered the gods by saying this.

The NP called the pharmacy, and my wife and I went over to pick up scripts for the new medications I'd be on. My world came full circle when I ran into a patient on our way through the store. It was the dad of the three-month-old baby I had performed a lumbar puncture on. To him, I was still "Doc," but I knew I had become the patient. It was hard to wrap my head around the circumstances.

Maureen and I had our days. Thankfully, we took turns. My head spun with worry. *Why me? I've treated hundreds of people. I am the only person I know with this specific condition.* I worried that I had passed a predisposition to this disease along to the kids. I worried about finances. Did we have enough for college? I was scared about how long I would live. Would I be able to provide enough for my family? Would we have enough to live on? Should I take my own life? Make it easier for my family? I sobbed intermittently.

And then, suddenly, we were very, very busy. We met with our lawyer; our friend, a CPA; and our financial planner. We went to medical appointments.

And then I had a heart-to-heart with my business partners. They were shocked and overwhelmed by the diagnosis. I had done pretty much everything. They were going to have to learn and then divvy up the responsibilities. There were time-sensitive tasks to complete, not the least of which was telling my patients that I would no longer be their doc. I wrote a brief note that went out to my caseload. It was emotionally draining, but there was no way around it. I had to give up my practice.

But it wasn't just being a doc. The practice was my baby. We had created a community. In the blink of an eye, something that I had built was gone. I had put so much into this and now I would no longer be there. My work had been a mistress who wouldn't be denied, but that was the cost of practicing the way I wanted. I was the soul of the place. I set the tone. I nurtured it.

I stayed on as a consultant to transition the business to the partners. I stopped driving as soon as I received the diagnosis. Though I had had no issues driving, this needed to be done. I gave it up willingly, just like I had my medical licenses. It was the right thing to do.

We initially chose to tell only those who needed to know and a handful of friends, who were unwavering in their support of us. We waited a month or so, until school was out, to tell the kids. During the year that followed, we spent time with them, with each other, and with close friends. We toiled long days on physical tasks—yard work, cleaning years' worth of collected items in the garage and the cellar, chopping wood, sledgehammering stone structures on the property—all in the hope of distracting ourselves from torturous thoughts. It was cathartic. We enjoyed nightly cocktails, cooked together, went on hikes and day trips, had lots of date nights, remembered our past, and counted our blessings.

Our close friends kept our confidence, and we were grateful for the gift of time to process. We are private people. We were allowed a year to wrap our heads around this nightmare before we were ready to be there to support our friends and extended family. This gave me time to finally reach the point where I had generally made peace with my lot in life. I was able to support those around me or tell them to get over themselves if they were getting too dramatic. It was what it was.

I received lots of cards from my patients. Every time I went into the practice, my office manager would hand me a stack of them. It would humble me to see who took the time to write thoughtful notes of good wishes, who sent kind gifts like books and Mass cards, and who asked my partners to let me know they were thinking of me. It meant a lot. During my visits at the practice, I often ran into my patients in the hallway. They cried; they missed me, they said. It was hard not to cry with them.

6

Life After Diagnosis

I never know what is going to happen day to day. Slowly, a combination of things has limited what I can do, unless someone is with me, and that has caused frustration. I had hopes of volunteering. I thought, *I can still do stuff. I can still help people.*

As far as the tests in the neurology office, it was frustrating—and demeaning—to do them over and over again. The tests took forever to complete, and they were not providing any new information. We knew I had difficulty drawing and writing. We knew I had difficulty with words. We knew I had trouble multitasking. Why did we need to rub it in?

Recently, I have been experiencing more symptoms of aphasia—trouble with talking, finding the right words. I have the pleasure of not being able to remember things that were said just moments before. This issue is such that I know what I want to say, but I can't get the words out. Or I think I've said the words, but I leave big gaps in my sentences. Sometimes I talk and work around the word or the thought, and it buys me time to make the connection for people I'm talking with. Sometimes I get "The Look" that makes it clear that though I know what I just said, people aren't understanding me. When they ask me to repeat what I said, they're too slow and then I can't recall it anymore. They are generally well-meaning people; they just can't understand me.

Talking is hard, but just give me a couple of characters, hints, I can get the words going again. I rarely pick up the phone because if someone isn't there to help, it doesn't go well. If I'm calm, if I'm warmed up, if I'm talking to someone I know, I do better. It takes a lot of trust. But there are times when it's just easier to listen. In one way or another, the aphasia determines how much you're going to be able to talk. As a species, we've evolved to use communication to get emotions across to each other. This advanced skill is how we gather, how we form groups, how we choose a mate, how we make connections. It's how we express our feelings, like "I don't like you" or "I'm having a bad day."

Communication doesn't have to be words. It could be music, it could be a look, a drawing, a gesture, a hand hold. We find a way. Nature finds a way. If you can talk, you're all set, but if you can't, there are ways to get around it. But all of these can be affected by aphasia. The worst thing is not being able to express what you want. Either you can't find the words or someone else can't understand you. Frustration is to be expected in any circumstance like this. We are human. There's a need to connect.

There are days when it gets really unnerving. I lose part of what I need or want. I'm trying to find a word and I can't. At work, I was the communication guy, the face of the company, but I took my functioning for granted. Back then, I was at full function, but now, I notice my hesitation and increased effort. It's extremely upsetting when I can't find the words. I get frustrated at the person I'm talking with. *Don't you get it? Don't you understand what I'm trying to tell you?* When I hear it in my head and when I say it, it sounds clear the majority of the time. There are times when people don't understand how hard it is to get those words, that emotion across. And when they realize I want to talk, the moment is gone. The thought is lost, I've moved on, I'm no longer able to share the emotion. That's how connections are lost. Listening indicates a desire, a measure of care, of concern, of selflessness, of support. If someone is showing that they cannot listen, it's hard to want to maintain that emotional connection. Thankfully, we have friends who get it, who are patient.

It takes trial and error, on both sides of the conversation. Sometimes success happens by just trying. Sometimes that might mean encouraging someone to sit and listen and not talk. For a person with aphasia, that trying might be advocating for themselves by gesturing that they want to add to the conversation but need to break in and have people listen. I want to talk. I've got one shot, just one. People don't listen. They talk fast with few breaks.

In addition to the aphasia, for a brief period of time, just before I received my diagnosis, I saw random faces. I thought it was interesting. They popped up on my right side and lasted only a split second. A cowboy, a little boy, a young woman—detailed, sharp, distinct, sepia colored. They all had neutral expressions and they looked right at me. I saw the deep wrinkles in the cowboy's face, his old, thick skin, his dusty hat. The little boy had dark hair that swept across his forehead. The young woman had light hair, shoulder length. I thought, *What was that? That was wild.* It didn't bother me. I told myself it's not real: clear as day, but fleeting. The EEG showed I was having increased electrical activity in the area of the brain associated with migraines with aura. I was started on a very low dose of antiseizure meds, and the faces went away the next day.

I also have trouble seeing things correctly. The table will be slanted or bowed, to the point that I lurch forward to catch plates before they slide off onto the floor. The barstool will be tipped, and I can't figure out how to start to safely sit on it. I put down my coffee cup on its side. I've been stymied and ultimately defeated by forks. My nemeses: mirrors, yoga, rights and lefts, playing pool, seatbelts. The pavement is uneven and it looks like a gulley runs through it. I search for things that are right in front of me. Things that are moving are easier to see.

Reading has become more difficult. When this started, words and numbers would interchange, or get squished. One time, I watched as a written capital *A* turned ninety degrees on the paper in front of me. I can no longer read more than a short string of words. I would jump sentences in a paragraph. I would slide a slip of paper down the page one line at a time to read the rows of numbers on a bank statement. I would read the first word in a sentence and, when I looked at the second word, the first word was disappearing.

On occasions, I've experienced a visual illusion that the room was stretching out in front of me. Everything was moving away very slowly. The first time it happened, I didn't know where I was as I walked down a seemingly narrow path. I was wigged out. I thought I was losing my mind. It's usually worse at night. With time, I have learned to talk myself through this visual phenomenon. *It's not real.* It no longer scares me, but it's still weird. I tell my wife, and she stays with me as I patiently wait for the room to come back to normal. Finding the right amount of light is essential. A little light helps, but not too much, because then the glare causes all the solid surfaces in my view to become blindingly shiny. Floors, countertops, door handles, picture frames, windows, utensils, a random pen lying on the table all become hard to look at when the light catches them at just the right angle.

There are many new experiences and emotions to navigate. I tread slowly on stairs. The handrail is essential. I find the top step and gauge the time and footfall distance as I walk down familiar steps. On new stairs, I turn my foot sideways on each stair. I don't like to eat in front of someone who isn't a friend. Sometimes it helps to close my eyes and take a break from all the visual noise. If we are in Target or the supermarket, I sometimes walk right by my wife. At other times, if I can't see her, it's as if she's not there, and I get lost. Not that long ago I was running around being helpful; now I think probably 80 percent of the time, the focus is on keeping me safe and making sure I don't get lost.

Memory is a funny thing. Random memories flow into my consciousness. It's a wonder to me that most days, I have trouble following instructions with more than one step, or remembering what I meant to do when I walked outside. But I remember events from decades ago with such clarity and detail. I think of songs: songs from my childhood, prom songs that I danced to with my wife, songs from college. I think of food—weird combinations, bad pie. My memories are solid, varied, palpable. I can pluck myself out of the here and now and immediately be in my childhood.

I recall visiting my great-grandmother in the old folks home. We could see it from our house, and we would walk over. It smelled like stale air. She was nice and she gave us candy. I would ask her to sing to us. I always asked for the same song, "The Animal Fair." She sang all the verses. I didn't realize how long it was until I looked it up recently. It was so kind of her to sing it every time. It resonates in my mind now, the part about "The monk, the monk, the monk, the monk." I loved it.

Teale Square Pub was a tavern frequented by college students. We hung out there over the years when we had a special occasion to celebrate. Senior week was one of those times. Our gang of five got together to sign up for karaoke as a band. We picked our outfits based on our limited college budget—white undershirts and jeans. Our song was "Crazy Little Thing Called Love," by Queen. I was the lead singer. I was excited; I had waited a long time to do this. At a recent gathering of the five, why was it me, the guy with Alzheimer's, who alone recalled the event? The brain is an amazing, funny thing.

As a student just out of college, some friends and I were invited to a Russian social club. Lots of old men, lots of vodka, lots of dancing. Perhaps my friends were under the influence of shots at the time, but again, years later, I was the only one who remembered the song, "Akh Odessa," that the old men were belting out in the club.

I was probably around five. I was staying with my grandmother, whom I adored. The antics of her first three children, rambunctious boys, taught her to be blunt and no nonsense. However, she also had a wicked sense of humor and was extremely kind. One time, she told me what we were having for lunch: deviled ham. She was good enough to ask what I wanted with it. I did not have a huge repertoire of lunch preferences at the age of five, so peanut butter was my go-to. She assessed me for a moment, then gave a sassy "okay" and headed to the pantry to make the weird sandwich for her strange little towheaded grandson. It turned out to be delicious—a perfect combination of sweet and salty, creamy and gritty, on spongy white bread. And I can taste it my memory, as if I were back in her kitchen.

I was again at my grandmother's house, but this time a bit older, maybe ten. It was late spring and she had made a pie for dessert. It looked delicious, with a beautiful lattice top with pink filling exposed in the spaces. Rhubarb. I asked if I could have some. She cut me a big piece and gently placed the plate in front of me. Delighted at this treat, I took my first bite. I chewed once. I don't know if I was more horrified at the tart mass that was in my mouth, or the false advertising. I squinted as my eyes began to water from the sting. I stopped chewing, but that made my tongue tingle even more. As my grandmother sat looking at me from across the table, this person I adored, I slowly resumed chewing. I swallowed hard, gulping for air in the hope of cleansing my palate. I rested a moment and put my fork down. My grandmother folded her arms and slowly leaned in toward me.

"You asked for a piece of pie. You will eat it. We do not waste food in this house."

I nodded and ate the pie that was so tart it curled my tongue. Later, I would find out she had tried a piece herself after I left for the day and threw the whole thing into the trash.

I think about how the brain works all the time. It's fascinating. One particular guy I worked with was a good example of this. I was the medical director for a local skilled-nursing facility. A new gentleman moved onto the Alzheimer's unit. He was settling in. There were a few things to wrap our heads around to make sure he was content and safe. He was a wanderer, which was not uncommon. He was up all night, assessing, looking into rooms, picking things up off the floor, going into the nurses' station. He was nonverbal, but pleasant. He really seemed to be purposeful and driven, but he was exhausted during the day. The staff was, of course, accustomed to having folks move around at odd hours, but we still wanted to know if there was a reason he was so consistently up at night.

We had the initial family meeting for planning his care. His kids had questions. Why was their dad still walking around? They were concerned about his wandering at night. Weren't we going to do something about that? The conversation turned to their father's job. It turns out he had worked as a night watchman, so it made sense that he was up all night. Even though he had been retired for years, in his mind, he was back to working. We supported him in doing what he needed to do. We also discussed his prior hobbies. He played the cornet. He couldn't converse, didn't go to activities during the day, didn't interact with other residents. He didn't even engage with his family that much. But he picked up that horn and went up and down the scales effortlessly. He played songs from memory. It was amazing. It ended up being so enjoyable for him that it was used as a behavioral technique to calm him down when he was anxious. It was perfect.

PART 2

Maureen

7

Younger-Onset Alzheimer's Disease: The Devil You Don't Know

A fifty-one-year-old woman who was experiencing confusion and delirium was brought to the hospital for an evaluation. She never returned home, spending the next five years in the hospital. It was the early 1900s. Back in the day, that was standard practice. Upon her death, her original psychiatrist was granted permission to study her brain. The doctor found physical anomalies normally seen in brains of folks decades older than his patient, Auguste D. The doctor's name was Alois Alzheimer, and he had just identified the condition that would come to bear his name. If she were a patient in the present day, Auguste D. would be diagnosed as having YOAD.

Alzheimer's disease (AD) is a condition in which there is a breakdown in the functioning of different parts of the brain. In a nutshell, for our body or mind to do anything, essential messages must be sent all around the brain via neurons, or nerve cells. These messages include any thoughts or directives. "I think I want sushi tonight," or "I hear a cat," or "Scratch your head. There's an itch above your right ear" are all sent as impulses by neurons. The system of transmission is from neuron to neuron, connecting one area of the brain to another. We make new connections as we need them to form new messages.

We could think of this system of communication as a complex transportation map of a major metropolitan area. There are roads, trains, walking paths, maybe some ferries. If you have an appointment across town, you have lots of options to get there. The majority of the time, you will probably choose to take the quickest, most direct route. Neurons like to do this too. Thoughts and actions come so easily that you often don't have to think about them: "Stop at the red light," "I'm from Massachusetts," "My friend's name is Bob," and the like.

Sometimes, thoughts and actions take a little longer. Think of this as a detour, or maybe the train broke down and now you must get on a bus. You will still get to your destination, but it's going to take a little longer than you thought. You might encounter this when you are trying to locate information in your brain that you haven't used in a while. Let's say you go to your high school reunion. *What was the name of my lab partner in physics class?* you wonder. She's right over there, and you'd like to say hello. Your brain begins a search, activating neurons in many different directions, checking any reasonable leads that are associated with this person, including memories from that period of time, like recalling the physics lab, any mutual friends, or a personal attribute. Eventually, you have your a-ha moment when her name pops into your head. *Of course, Suzie Q!* How could you have forgotten?

With Alzheimer's disease, the process of getting information or directives from one area of the brain to another slowly breaks down. Rather than a detour, it might be a major snowstorm that you are facing, and many roads are closed or impassable. You may get to your destination eventually, but it will take much more effort on your part to find a path to get there. A person with Alzheimer's might find the ability to read words more and more challenging, until recognizing letters may become a task that can no longer be completed. It may be that someone loses the ability to coordinate the use of a knife and fork to cut food. The old pathways are broken, but new pathways have not been created.

Most people have a vision of folks with Alzheimer's disease. Maybe they see someone who is old; maybe they envision someone who repeatedly asks questions and forgets who family members are; maybe they think of someone who wanders around or collects things. On a cellular level, Later-Onset Alzheimer's Disease (LOAD) and YOAD have a common thread. They seem to be caused by the same disruptions in cell structure and function. But that's where the similarities end. Forget everything you have ever known about the disease. This is not your grandfather's Alzheimer's.

Shocking as it might be, you could be working right next to someone who has Alzheimer's. Your kid's roommate at college might have a parent going through this. Do you go to the gym, or are you in a running club? It wouldn't be out of the realm of possibility to see someone with Alzheimer's there too. This can be a prime-of-life condition, a diagnosis that affects people when they are hitting their strides. Medically speaking, YOAD (also known as early-onset Alzheimer's disease) is Alzheimer's-type dementia diagnosed in people younger than sixty-five. However, symptoms usually begin when someone is in their forties or fifties and, in some rare cases, have been seen in people as young as their thirties.

This condition causes disruption in every aspect of living. Thoughts can run rampant. Many worries are practical: You've worked hard to get promoted. Can you still do your job? You have a decade to go before even thinking about retirement. What about your pension? Your house isn't paid off yet. You carry the health insurance. Your condo has three flights of stairs. Your relationship with your partner is already brittle. You are taking care of an elderly parent. You live in a rural setting and need to drive to town to get anything. You are a single parent, and your kid wants to go to college. The sheer number of concerns and the enormity of the situation is almost too much to digest.

There are very few who get a warning shot across the bow. According to researchers, 90 to 95 percent of all cases of YOAD are sporadic, meaning it is rare to have a genetic predisposition for getting this disease. In contrast, LOAD, in which people are diagnosed after the age of sixty-five, does have identified gene variations that indicate a higher risk of being passed down to the next generation. While there is ongoing research and much speculation as to root causes of YOAD, to date, medicine has not been able to definitively identify what to avoid, what to increase, or how to change our lives to lower the chances of being diagnosed with this condition, nor are there any telltale signs that one may eventually develop it. It comes out of left field.

The actual diagnosis of YOAD is also particularly tricky. Symptoms differ vastly compared with traditional amnestic-type AD, and the same symptoms can often be attributed to other factors. Difficulty with speech can be chalked up to multitasking, or to stress from work, parenting, maintaining relationships, or caring for parents or relatives. Visual-perceptual difficulties usually result in a trip to the optometrist; it's probably about time to get reading glasses. That achiness you feel in your muscles? Did the weekend of yardwork catch up with you? Are you pushing the miles too hard training for that half-marathon? Or are you just getting older, and things are starting to fall apart? When your thinking feels just a little slower or you make a rookie mistake, you might wonder if those multiple trips to the bathroom in the night are affecting your sleep.

It's not just the average person who might be stumped by these symptoms. In one study, researchers found an increased wait time for diagnosis of YOAD compared with that of late-onset Alzheimer's disease. The average time from initial visit with primary care to eventual diagnosis of YOAD at the hospital was about two years. The list of differential diagnoses that encompass symptoms of YOAD is lengthy. In the medical world, common things are common and rare things are rare. It usually makes sense to start with simple possibilities and move on from that point. It's hard to believe someone in the prime of their life is fighting Alzheimer's. "It must be something else."

On a cellular level, current research has identified two major players that seem to be involved in the Alzheimer's disease process. Both are proteins found in the brain. One is called tau and another is called amyloid-beta. These proteins actively support the function of the brain and neurons. Tau is located inside nerve cells and looks something like a wet piece of spaghetti. It sits across and tucked between structures that resemble hollow ears of corn with kernels arranged in a spiral. The spiral structure is called a microtubule, a transport tunnel for materials needed for cell function. The tau acts to provide dynamic stability. In folks with Alzheimer's, tau pieces break off the microtubule and then fold in on themselves, sticking together like pieces of Scotch tape. Multiple pieces of sloughed-off tau often bind together; these are referred to as "tangles." As a result, the tangles can block the microtubule passageways, inhibiting the flow of materials. In addition, without the aid of the tau to hold them together, the tiny beads of the microtubule spiral structure begin to separate, essentially breaking down the tunnel.

Amyloid-beta is the other protein that has been implicated in AD pathology. In healthy brains, amyloid seems to play an important role in neuron health. This protein is thought to work as a security guard to keep the brain safe from any nefarious characters trying to enter and as a medic to help heal the brain from insult and injury. In the disease-free process, amyloid naturally ages, breaks apart, and is cleared away effectively by the body. In the degenerative process of AD, however, these protein fragments stay in the brain and collect in the space around and between the neurons. Amyloid-beta fragments can clump together, forming bundles called plaques. These plaques and fragments disrupt the functioning of the neurons and can eventually cause the death of the nerve cell.

One study has estimated the prevalence of people living with some sort of young onset dementia as 3.9 million people world-wide, with approximately 200,000 of those living in the U.S. This research included diagnoses of vascular dementia and frontotem-poral degeneration (FTD), as well as YOAD. This number is also suspected to be greatly underestimated due to lack of comprehen-sive data, especially information from lower-income nations and on people on the younger end of the diagnostic age range. Care planning and increased disease awareness would benefit from ac-curate data.

A diagnosis of YOAD does not only carry the burdens of planning for the future. The day-to-day emotional roller coaster is exhausting. Unlike with an amnestic-type dementia, folks with YOAD have an awareness of the disease process and how it impacts their lives. There is no blissfully unaware, happily confused state, especially in the early stages. This a frustrating, mentally taxing condition that continues to get worse. With this younger population, depression and anxiety are common. It is crucial for family, friends, and anyone else caring for the person to be acutely aware of this risk and be proactive about treatment and strategies. One of the most important points to consider with YOAD is that a person's sense of self often remains the same for quite a long period of time. Personality, sense of humor, work ethic, and self-identity are still apparent. Tapping into these constants can help to ensure a link to normalcy and routine, and help stabilize emotional health.

Maintaining relationships with old friends is helpful, but so is finding new acquaintances who know from their own experience what you are going through. This might happen through joining a support group, attending a lecture on YOAD, being part of a research study, or chatting it up with someone in the waiting room when you go to see your neurologist. Many times, people feel quite isolated because they do not know anyone else with this condition. While there are close to four million people in the world with some type of young-onset dementia, YOAD is considered a rare disease, comprising only 5 to 6 percent of all AD diagnoses. It's easy to feel like you are one in a million, and not in a good way.

The younger-onset form of AD generally impacts very different areas of the brain than Later-Onset Alzheimer's. The tau tangles and amyloid-beta plaques are present in both versions, but beyond that, the similarities seem to end. The neighborhoods of the brain impacted in YOAD tend to produce difficulties in functioning that in no way appear to be typical AD. Rather, it often comes as a surprise to many to learn that the strange-yet-common sequelae described in the upcoming chapters are what folks with YOAD encounter on a day-to-day basis. These can be confusing, frustrating, and sometimes just plain scary. Knowledge is power; the next few chapters aim to shed light on some of these characteristic symptoms to allow for some emotional, mental, and physical preparation. The accompanying strategies may also give a measure of control over a situation that, at times, can seem to be running amok.

8

Life Comes at You Fast

Strange occurrences began to happen around our house. I would find plates teetering on the edge of the counter, cups lying on their sides. One of our kids noted that Dad looked like he was doing Pilates when eating. Dan started to feel slightly carsick as a passenger, and sometimes he had to take a break from watching a movie.

While we initially found it hard to find a common thread connecting these phenomena, the diagnosis of YOAD made it clear that these were not out-of-the-ordinary experiences and that they were indeed linked.

The temporal and parietal lobes are parts of the brain often targeted by amyloid-beta plaques and tau tangles. The temporal lobes are on either side of your head, at about the level of your ears, and are mainly responsible for language. The parietal lobes, which are on the top of your head, about where your headphone strap would rest, are essential to collecting sensory information from different areas of the brain so you can move your body through your environment. They help you judge the distance and location of objects and coordinate accuracy and speed of movement of your body. Your fully functioning parietal lobes, for example, are an important factor in allowing you to effortlessly reach out, grasp, and hold a glass of water, then bring it to your mouth to drink.

The younger-onset type of Alzheimer's has been referred to by many names. One of these is "the visual variant" of the disease and, as one can imagine, it affects every part of life. More than the acuity or sharpness of vision, YOAD affects the perception of what is seen. For Dan, paragraphs were hard to follow, as were rows of numbers on a spreadsheet; his eyes would automatically jump to the line below. At times, the words would seem to lose their spacing and become one big, long word. Other times, the words and numbers would dance around the page, and sometimes they would disappear altogether. Dan went for his eye exam, partly for a recommendation on reading glasses, but partly because things just "looked different." Turns out he could see those distance eye-chart letters clearly, and the closer ones required only a weak bump in diopter strength. The issue was that his brain was not interpreting visual information easily. Our super-savvy ophthalmologist was able to tease out the issue of acuity versus perception by feeding Dan one letter at a time. By blocking the rest of the visual information, he reduced the "visual clutter," and Dan's brain was able to concentrate on one item at a time. Knowing this information didn't make the situation any easier to digest, but it was helpful to know why it was happening. Once we knew, we could adapt.

I began to take a close look around our house. What might be a potential barrier for Dan? There were definitely changes we could make to improve the ease and success of doing normal, everyday things. Nothing big. We wanted the house to be accessible and safe, but we also wanted it to still feel like home. Here are a few small changes that made a big difference:

- **Light it up like a Christmas tree.** There were pockets of uneven light in some of our rooms. Adding additional table or floor lamps on the perimeter of each room filled in the gaps. Dark spaces like the cellar and garage needed additional overhead lighting. We swapped our single 60-watt bulb for a bright LED fixture with adjustable panels. You can find ones that will screw into the existing electrical fixture and have ample light in seconds.

- **Leave the light on for me.** Having a path of light to follow through the house or to greet you when you enter is extremely welcoming. Sometimes light switches are hard to find in low light, so having some lights come on at dusk avoids the trouble of running around preparing for the night. Old-fashioned timers rigged up to a lamp can help, but your smart home or some high-tech options also make this an easy feat. A night-light or lamp left on can help light the path to the bathroom. Light-up switches can also replace existing pole switches and provide a nice little beacon.

- **Clear the area.** Keeping your space clear both physically and visually is priceless. Accessible paths into and around the house are needed for safety. Puppy toys, accent furniture, random backpacks, and shoes on the floor are all liable to cause a fall. Objects won't necessarily be seen by someone with YOAD, even though they may look obvious to others. Visual clutter is also an issue. We had a decorative basket on top of the toilet tank. It had pine cones in it. It was super cute, but it ended up being a huge visual distraction and made that part of Dan's day more difficult, so it was removed. Not worth it. If the table you eat at can be uncluttered and uncrowded, it will make dinner easier. Remove extraneous items, like the salt and pepper shakers, the napkin holder, or your keys. Having one thing to concentrate on at a time helps your brain to take a bit of a mental breather.

• **Make dinner a colorful affair.** We eat a lot of yellow food. This was a very strange observation I made in the first few months after Dan's diagnosis. Pineapple, omelets, quiche, cheese, and bananas were often on the menu. And there were other foods that were in the same color family, maybe ochre or beige: chicken, crackers, burrito wraps, Dan's favorite bakery cinnamon buns. The issue was not the food, but the plates. Dan and I had excitedly packed up our thirty-year-old white plates and gifted them to one of our kids, who was moving into their first apartment. We spent time looking over our options and finally settled on some beautiful, sturdy, big—and yellow—plates. Who knew? These days, yellow food goes on the blue tapas-sized plates or in the little glass Pyrex custard dishes. The color contrast makes meal times go more smoothly.

• **Take it slow.** Not all helpful changes require moving furniture. One very useful technique takes into account the fact that processing information takes time and effort. For someone with YOAD, greater concentration and longer processing time is the norm. While we may think of processing difficulties in terms of verbal skill, visual-perceptual processing is also impacted in significant ways. I've had clients report increased use of applying the "pretend brake" as a passenger. They've felt more uneasy with cars merging in front of them on the highway, as though they swerved in too quickly, narrowly avoiding an accident.

Similarly, just handing Dan a glass of water can cause him to rapidly withdraw backward, with a look of shock. With this diagnosis, life is literally coming at you fast. The eyes can see the object in view, but the brain needs just a little bit more time to figure out which direction the object is coming from and how soon it will arrive. Understanding this phenomenon can lead to better days. Fast movement leads to stress and visual fatigue; slower movement allows for success with completing a given task. Presenting that yellow dinner plate happens very slowly now, and it also comes with a verbal warning that it is on its way into Dan's visual field. My rapid movements from one task to the next have slowed significantly, because they make Dan dizzy. I had to coach myself to reduce my speed and sometimes just plain stop. It isn't intuitive for me, but I've come to realize how helpful it is for Dan, so I try my best.

As if YOAD weren't rare enough, there is sometimes a risk of developing an associated disorder called posterior cortical atrophy (PCA). It's a complex array of fascinating yet debilitating neuro-logical irregularities which equates to visual processing deficits on steroids. Research into this disease is ongoing and much is still unknown. While AD is the most common underlying diagnosis, other diseases can also cause PCA. There is much underreporting and misdiagnosing that occurs. Folks with PCA don't present with typical dementia symptoms and are commonly referred to ophthal-mology or optometry, as the signs point to an issue with optical functioning, not cognitive abilities. The true issue is due to plaques in the parietal and/or occipital lobes that hamper perceptual skills. The brain just can't make heads or tails out of some of what it is perceiving and, in some cases, won't perceive things at all.

Back in OT school, we learned about rare phenomena caused by neurological diseases. They were almost too far-fetched to be-lieve. We saw old black-and-white clinic photos in our textbooks—patients attempting simple movements without success, writing and clock-drawing samples with strange deviations from the norm. Most of us never expected to see these in our own practice. I must say I was stunned when one of my first clients literally did not eat half of what was on their plate because they didn't "see" it. Such visual-perceptual issues shocked me less and less as I worked in the field. They came with the territory when folks were recovering from strokes and brain injuries.

But life is always surprising. The manifestations of PCA can be truly wild. There are a number of specific skill deficits that can be attributed to this disease, and they all have the potential for significant impact on daily life:

- difficulty working with numbers to complete calculations (acalculia)

- inability to identify the left side of your body from your right (left-right disorientation)

- inability to tell which finger was touched without looking (finger agnosia)

- inability to write your independent thoughts or a statement dictated to you (agraphia)

- difficulty moving your eyes smoothly in a horizontal plane to track or locate an object (ocularmotor apraxia)

- problems with accurately reaching out to voluntarily grasp an object (optic ataxia)

- inability to perceive more than one object at a time in a setting where there are many objects (simultanagnosia)

The first four symptoms are collectively known as the rare disorder Gerstmann syndrome. The last three symptoms make up Balint syndrome, another type of unusual diagnosis. Any one symptom would be a challenge; having to battle a number of these issues while performing your job, taking care of your family, or just plain living your life is daunting. It really requires good communication, lots of support, and some trial and error to come

up with a system for success when presented with these challenges.

While not part of one of the named syndromes above, difficulty with reading or perceiving words (alexia) can occur in varying
degrees with PCA. Sometimes the words get squished together on
the page, or sentences in a paragraph can meld together. Sometimes letters dance around on the page, or they might disappear
altogether.

Motor issues are also a common occurrence with PCA. Folks
might feel an electrical shock, a jerk or push, or a quick tightness
in a muscle group. This is referred to as myoclonus, and it can be
distracting at best, debilitating at worst. It can wake you up at
night; it can force you to stop and catch your breath. It can come
on in an instant and go away just as quickly. This was one of the
consistent issues Dan had prior to getting his formal YOAD diagnosis, and we assumed it was from training for his big birthday
half-marathon. Until we started to put all of the pieces together,
we didn't realize what we had in front of us.

Longer-lasting tightness in a muscle group can also be an issue
in folks with PCA. This increased level of muscle tone is known as
spasticity. The arm on one side might be held in a slightly bent
position at rest, or someone's gait might be marginally off due to
increased tightness in the muscles of one part of the leg. It might
seem like the arm is "catching on something" when you try and
move it.

Finally, there is one more major brain-dictated motor phenomenon that occurs commonly with PCA: apraxia. Ideomotor apraxia
is quite common with PCA and can be observed when someone
tries to physically perform a familiar activity. It becomes readily
apparent that they are unable to figure out how to motor-plan to
actually do the task. The issue is not due to volition, nor is there
difficulty with muscle coordination, strength, or range of motion.
The task at hand most likely has been learned or overlearned,

practiced and perfected in the past. And, if asked to perform the task, the issue is not related to understanding directions. The brain just cannot figure out how to plan, initiate, and sequence the steps to do the job. Folks can become frozen in their tracks, losing their place or rhythm or can have difficulty even moving from the start.

Ideomotor apraxia, if present when performing one activity, most often will bleed into other tasks as well. And even the most mundane, effortless tasks can take a hit. Bit by bit, the flow starts to get interrupted, and it becomes more and more difficult to complete the task. One ability commonly affected by apraxia is using utensils. Cutting food with a knife and fork is quite a high-level, coordinated skill. If presented with these utensils, someone with PCA may examine them or expend tremendous effort in trying to wield them, but in the end, may not be able to successfully coordinate the motor movements to cut their food.

Dressing apraxia is also seen regularly in folks with PCA. The complex abilities required to find a shirt sleeve, thread a belt through the carriers, engage a separated zipper, or tie a shoe are truly mind-boggling. Finding work-arounds is essential to maintaining dignity and independence. There are myriad options for more user-friendly clothing and techniques to make these activities easier. Enlisting the help of an occupational therapist can go a long way in facilitating the success of these activities.

Lastly, consider that complex daily activities, including dressing, bathing, cooking, and using technology, all become that much more challenging given that people with PCA will often have a triple threat of perceptual disturbances, muscle issues, and ideomotor apraxia. Add to that the progressive nature of the disease, awareness of symptoms on the part of the person with PCA, and the oftentimes accompanying anxiety and depression, and daily life can be challenging at each turn.

So what can help? First, knowing there is a scientific reason for what is going on is a good place to start. Folks aren't making this stuff up. That helps both the person with PCA and those who know and love them. It takes the drama out of the scenario.

Talking about what is going on is also eye-opening, humbling, and can create an opportunity for connection. Feeling enough trust to share and finding a compassionate enough soul to listen can be a monumental task. If that happens, though, all manner of communication can occur. Can you discuss the frustration you might feel when you can't reason out how to do something you'd done every day of your life? Could you talk about how frightening it is to look across the room and see it slowly stretch out in front of you? It might make the whole experience a little less bizarre. It might allow you to have company during the process. Will talking about the muscle tightness that comes over you in waves allow you to problem solve with a partner, to see if there is a pattern, and then, a solution?

Having someone who understands, or at the very least, listens can make a huge impact. That someone could be anyone of your choosing. I've seen folks make connections with others in their support groups. Maybe you are fortunate to have a caring doctor, health-care provider, or therapist. Maybe there is a family member or friend you can confide in. For care partners, this communication serves to maintain a bond, to preserve some of "the before." But it also just helps us feel not as useless. Have the shared experience—laugh, cry, live to tell the tale. Make the connection.

There have been specific approaches that have made life a little easier. Some were realized through hard-fought trial and error, others were stumbled upon. Some techniques were useful for a time, but then were abandoned for a better option or because, for any number of reasons, they no longer worked. And, truly, things can change moment to moment. What might work one day—or one hour—simply doesn't work the next. Some of these ideas might be of help.

Eating. Present one utensil for a meal. That means food might need to be prepped a bit. Cutting down on options sends a clear message that this one utensil is what you can use. Cups may work better than mugs as the handle can be visually distracting or pose a challenge for motor planning. Shorter cups and glasses can help decrease the angle needed to drink. Hand-held foods, like pizza, tacos, gyros, or paninis are nice options for maintaining dignity, encouraging independence, and having shared meal experiences with others.

Errands. Dan and I are a really sappy couple, holding hands wherever we've gone since we first started dating. This helps tremendously while we are shopping, walking through the supermarket, or even maneuvering around the airport. It gives Dan reassurance on the periphery of his visual field and keeps him from losing me. We've also done the "flank" or "follow" techniques. Dan can be put back on track if I walk next to him and physically coax him back to center. I've also walked in front of him so he has a visual target in sight.

Activities of daily living (ADLs). Everyday, we make this calculation: How much assistance is needed versus how much independence is appropriate? We consider it a big win in our house when we successfully anticipate hiccups and set tasks up for success. For judiciously chosen activities, simply written step-by-step directions have been helpful with ideomotor apraxia. "Do this, then this, then this." Practice makes better, success breeds success, and less is more. Some activities are considered "two putts." How can you make them easier? Lid off the deodorant and cap off the toothpaste, clothes laid out in the order they are put on, electric razor instead of standard safety razor and shaving cream, leaving the cereal box on the table instead of trying to find it in the pantry in the morning.

When your brain says you are seeing two of everything, simplifying whatever visual information you are receiving is necessary. It is also surprisingly easier to visually "catch" items that are moving rather than trying to locate a stationary object. I will often offer Dan one medication at a time, with a verbal cue when moving it within view so it can be tracked and picked up. I also keep in mind the color of the pill relative to the background where I place it. White pill on black napkin, red capsule on white countertop.

Home safety. As an OT, doing a safety evaluation and implementing recommendations are essential parts of the job—one I can honestly say always kept me up at night when I was treating patients. The responsibility weighed heavily on my mind, and things are no different now that I have the same responsibility here at home. Finding the secret sauce for perfect home safety and independence is a constant worry, especially with PCA. You could outfit your home with every safety device out there, but with this perceptual deficit, more is not necessarily better. Would it help to have a handrail in the bathroom, or would that just be more visually distracting and potentially cause a fall? Small rugs are usually a big no-no, but with PCA, you often need a visual target. Having a handrail on the stairs is a nonstarter; however, which side do you put it on? Sometimes a person's physically stronger side may also be the weaker side for their visual perception. Many folks with YOAD and PCA don't "see" things in plain sight, or they may completely disregard everything on one side. Lighting is also crucial. Consistent, even lighting can decrease shadows, make objects appear less fuzzy or distorted, and assist with creating clearly marked pathways.

An OT or physical therapist (PT) can be a valuable resource to consult about home safety. If someone is receiving home services, a home safety evaluation is often part of the team assessment, and specific recommendations can be made based on what the nurses and therapists feel might be helpful currently or in the future.

Mental and physical health. While addressing the unique issues that impact day-to-day functioning, it is also critical to maintain your health throughout this time. This is a long-term process, a marathon not a sprint, so having the ability to operate optimally is a plus. We've found a few methods to support this goal.

Creating daily or weekly routines is a helpful way to anticipate what's to come. It also allows your brain to expend a little less energy. When there is a familiar schedule, there is one less thing for you to consciously plan or worry about.

Exercise is medicine, be it in the form of working out or doing something active. It can give you a way to release energy, loosen up the muscle tightness, and maintain balance. Having a conversation with your MD about meds for myoclonus, getting a PT referral, and finding a stretching or gentle yoga program could be good ways to start.

Find meaningful activities to do for others. It's more difficult to feel bad about your situation when you are helping someone in need. Volunteer, assist a neighbor, donate to a worthy cause. Figure out how you can find purpose, be useful, and give of yourself.

Sometimes routine starts to become, well, routine. Changing things up can alter your perspective and provide a mental reset. Get out of Dodge, even if it's just taking a day trip, going for a walk on a new trail, or meeting up with a friend.

9

I Know What I Want to Say

Younger-Onset Alzheimer's disease finds root in the temporal lobes of the brain. This area is the hub of language, allowing you to speak and understand words. A hit to this region will often result in aphasia, or difficulty with communication, and it can take many forms. Folks with YOAD often have difficulty finding the words they are looking for. The words are in there, sometimes even on the tip of their tongue, but it's hard to pull them out. This disorder is called primary progressive aphasia (PPA); the logopenic variant of this condition (lvPPA) is the type usually seen in people with YOAD. The research team at the Mesulam Center at Northwestern University was the first to identify PPA as a distinct diagnosis and to separate it into its specific variants.

When aphasia occurs as a result of neurological trauma or stroke, the injury is initially worse after the event and then slowly stabilizes as the region begins to heal. With PPA, the communication difficulty is minimal at first and slowly gets worse. One common feature is circumlocution, or talking around the word you are missing. Sometimes this buys people time to actually locate the word they are looking for; sometimes it just helps to avoid a lapse in conversation by coming up with a word that's close to what they're looking for. Another common characteristic of PPA is called paraphasia. This may involve a change to a word's sound by substituting, adding, or transposing parts of a word. Instead of "bread," someone might say "pread," or "apple" comes out as "lapple." A paraphasia can also involve the meaning of a word, such as saying "bowl" for "plate" or "screwdriver" for "wrench." Sometimes the person will catch the altered word but just as often, the conversation will continue without correction.

When emotions run high, when fatigue is in play, or when there is physical discomfort, such as feeling chilly or too warm or having to use the bathroom, communication is affected. In these situations, words become tangled or repeated, or even just evaporate. Sometimes there is a feedback loop that occurs: One fragment of a thought or sentence may be repeated over and over as someone tries to communicate the next thought. Dan has always been a great storyteller, with a wealth of material from which to draw. He shares stories with excitement, joy, passion, a great deal of humor, and excellent comedic timing. Now it seems that this exuberance is bubbling over as Dan tells these stories, almost like he's riding down a hill on a bike and fighting hard to control the direction and speed.

Back when we were kids, there was a show on the Saturday morning lineup of cartoons called *Schoolhouse Rock*. The episodes were all designed to teach a concept, be it math, grammar, science, or even how a bill becomes a law. They were hugely entertaining and had catchy little songs that stuck with you. One of the grammar lessons had a stout and very agile train conductor walking over the cars of a train. The segment was called "Conjunction Junction," and, as advertised, it taught some of the possible ways to connect thoughts together with teeny words. Alzheimer's never

fails to surprise: For example, conjunctions are often what is repeated when an exciting story is being told. I can envision the
conductor landing on each train car roof: And. But. Or. So. And.
But. Or. So.

As a care partner, having ways to reliably communicate both
information and emotion is essential for day-to-day activities, for
everyone's mental health, and for continuing to support the relationship you had before this diagnosis. Trying out different techniques and approaches is helpful; not everyone is going to subscribe
to or benefit from every method. And while a technique might be
helpful in one situation or during a period of time, it may become
obsolete. Knowing that it's okay to ditch what isn't working can
help you move on to a different, more successful approach.

Some techniques and concepts that have been helpful for our
family include the following:

Be a reporter . . . but be efficient in your questioning.
The standard "who, what, when, where, why, how" will usually
get you the information you need to move the conversation
forward. "Twenty questions," however, is really difficult and can
often end up frustrating everyone. One party wants to easily
pass along information; the other party wants to easily grasp the
information. Too many unrelated questions can muddy the
waters and turn the conversation off topic. If the questions are
seemingly coming out of left field, the person telling the story
can also end up wondering if the other person is actually
listening.
Less is more. PPA is a difficulty with communication, which
means both getting information out and getting information in.
This is called expressive and receptive communication, respec-
tively. Peppering someone with questions to clarify or "help" is
not necessarily helpful. I often go by an 80-20 rule. Eighty percent of the time, Dan is given the opportunity to communicate,

and that includes time actively talking as well as finding the words in his head. I'll jump in when he is done making his thoughts known. It's a hard thing to do, especially for someone who likes to talk and who likes answers quickly. I can also say that rule adjusts to 95-5 on the rough days when expressing information is especially challenging. To ensure a person knows you are actively listening to what they are saying, verbally and nonverbally, a short statement—"Okay," "I'm listening," "Tell me more," and the like—is not terribly intrusive or distracting and can bolster rapport. Reassurance can also be provided by your facial expression, body language, or a touch. A nod or a smile goes a long way to support and encourage.

To receive information effectively, one first needs to be attending to the speaker. It helps to have a heads-up when someone wants to tell you something. I've told care partners that when a long sentence is spoken, someone with PPA may only get the middle part. A three-part sentence might be something like, "On Friday, I saw Mary at the store, and she said she got a new puppy." The first part of the sentence often ends up being the cue that someone is speaking to you: "I need to pay attention. Someone is going to tell me something." The person with PPA will now be able to hear the middle section, that you saw Mary at the store. The end of the sentence is often lost because it encompasses the period of time spent processing information—"Mary. Which Mary? Which store? Why is this important for me to know?"—and the news of the puppy will inevitably be a surprise later. To the speaker, the message is crystal clear, so it can be confusing and frustrating if this information doesn't get imparted.

With that being said, a heads-up in the form of a gesture (a gentle wave, eye contact, a smile) or a verbal cue ("Hi. I have something to tell you.") allows the conversation to start right away. Information will be easier to digest in smaller chunks.

Shorter sentences with breaks in between can be helpful. Lastly, less is more with volume as well. While we often speak in clipped sentences when we are raising our voices, the emotional tone can often obscure the true message; speaking in a low tone or even whispering is often better at catching attention and getting important thoughts across.

The Goldilocks Zone. We all have times when we are operating on all four cylinders. We can also recognize when we are hitting a wall. We all find our ability to function is affected by the conditions in and around us. Physical, mental, and emotional states, as well as the setting in which you are working all impact performance. Optimally, you would have your most important conversations and complete your most challenging work when you are in your "Goldilocks Zone," feeling awake, calm, and alert, physically rested, neither too hot nor too cold, no full bladder telling you to run to the bathroom, and in a welcoming state of mind to complete your task. This ideal state has a smaller window when PPA is involved. The same principles apply, but it becomes much more important to actively foster the ideal conditions to facilitate good communication. Also, circle back to critical information to ensure that the message sent was received accurately. Given the myriad variables that can affect communication, discrepancies can exist between what was said and what was heard. Correcting these quickly can stave off frustration, confusion, and misdirection.

Talk to yourself. As a care partner, it helps to be your own cheerleader when PPA is on the scene. Putting yourself in a positive place is essential but certainly easier said than done. Keeping your focus on trying to figure out the emotion in the message is important when the words don't seem to make sense. Having reminders for yourself always at the ready can help. Mantras like "They're not doing this on purpose," and "The word is in there; it's just filed in the wrong place," can redirect you to a better state. So can just taking a break and walking away. Go outside and play fetch with the dog, take a bathroom break, go check the mailbox, text a meme to a friend. It's okay to be mad at the PPA, the Alzheimer's, the loss. Giving a bit of daylight between you and the conversation can really allow you to regroup and come back to the situation with a renewed focus and less emotional baggage.

10

Sleeping on Your Feet

When Dan was a resident, he had some rough months on call. There would be nights when the pager would go off every half hour. He was so spent, he would sleep right through the incessant buzzing. I felt awful waking him up. When he was on call in the hospital, he slept in the residents' room when he could. It was harder to ignore the phone calls from the nurses' station, but not impossible. He came home after one particularly busy night and told me that, apparently, he had picked up the phone and, in his exhausted state, put it right down on the cradle, turned over, and gone back to sleep. The nurse ended up marching down the hall, opening the door to the residents' room, and turning on all the lights. He woke up then.

We've all been there. Sleeping on our feet. Maybe it was when you were working third shift or pulling an all-nighter cramming for an exam. Anyone with a newborn understands the utter fatigue that comes along with having to wake up and be functional every twenty minutes or so. Or you might have experienced this mental drain when training for a new job. Maybe it wasn't the physical exhaustion that caused you to be tired, but the fact that you had to focus so intently to retain new information that it caused your brain to say "uncle." In all of these instances, your brain knew what it wanted, and it wanted sleep.

With Alzheimer's, everything gets just a little bit harder. Understanding conversations takes more concentration. Finding the word you are looking for is akin to having a program constantly running in the background, eating up energy. Making sense of visual information you are receiving is a necessary but multifaceted process. You really do need to know where to put your foot on the next step, locate the food on your plate, and get dressed. These challenges happen all day long, concurrent with the other tasks in your daily life. They compete for your attention, your energy, and your patience. It is no wonder folks dealing with this condition often become completely drained. It's like bonking—suddenly running out of energy—during a run. Your brain just tells you to stop. There's nothing left to give. Accepting the reality of the increased energy demand can help put the need for some extra sleep into perspective. Power naps are a beautiful thing. So is snacking. Your brain needs fuel.

Alzheimer's doesn't take a day off, and as it progresses, it doesn't just cause fatigue, it disrupts the entire sleep-wake cycle by actually targeting the specific parts of the brain that regulate the process. The hypothalamus and its component parts tell your brain to power down for sleep and give you the signals to wake up again. Without this smooth regulation, bad things happen. Dysregulation due to neurodegenerative causes or trauma can cause a condition called secondary narcolepsy. Similar to its well-known cousin, secondary narcolepsy causes a person to fall asleep when they do not want to. They could be in the middle of a sentence or may have just sat down for a moment. While this is inconvenient for holding a conversation, the bigger issue is when dream states begin to intersect with reality. Secondary narcolepsy often comes with the burden of quickly falling into dreaming sleep. During this time, you may hear someone with this condition talking in their sleep or acting out their dreams. And because secondary narcolepsy also derails the system for waking up from these states, there is often a prolonged, fuzzy sense of surroundings and reality.

Your dream state might dictate your actions; I've worked with people who thought they were in the bathroom, when in actuality they were in the bedroom. When you look around, things seem to look familiar, but are a little off. It can become a stressful situation rapidly. It takes patience, finesse, and trust to prevent an escalation, or to right a situation that has already gone awry.

Consider this scenario: You wake up from a nap and a strange person is walking around your house. I do not think many folks would engage said stranger in conversation to explain their presence. The first reaction would likely be confusion, fear, or anger, and the immediate inclination would be to get the stranger out of your house. Your brain is still waking up and cannot recognize who or what is familiar, nor is it in any state to be convinced otherwise. Some techniques to help during the transition back to being fully awake can include the following:

> **Buy time.** If it takes increased time to wake up, then time is what they need. Don't ask lots of questions, don't flip all the lights on, keep the vibe in the room calm. A slow reorientation at their own pace, and perhaps some gentle cueing is a good approach.
> **Surrender control.** A person with a clear sense that something is out of the ordinary will want some measure of autonomy over the situation. Allow them to walk around to assess the situation and feel safe. Familiarity can help with righting the ship: a recognizable setting, background noise that they might be accustomed to, interacting with pets, seeing a neighbor,

talking with a family member. Having a communication station—a go-to place to find important information, like date, day of the week, a daily activity list, and who is home—can also be a good method for preserving someone's independence in gathering evidence. Give ample space and time for them to come to their own conclusions about whether they can let their guard down.

Don't correct. Giving seemingly conflicting information to someone already burdened with trying to make sense of a situation can derail it altogether. Answer questions with succinct answers using a matter-of-fact, nonconfrontational tone.

Talk to your provider. There are medications, vitamins, and supplements that can assist with regulation of the sleep-wake cycle and to tamp down increased anxiety. Have frank conversations with trained professionals who know the ins and outs of the diagnosis, best treatments, important considerations for safety, and, most importantly, is familiar with the person living with the diagnosis.

11

My Love

Alzheimer's has altered Dan's life in significant ways, touching every aspect of being. He is the living epitome of Sisyphus pushing a boulder up a mountain every day. It is a cruel sentence for someone so kind. While there are often moments and days that overwhelm and demoralize, I am always amazed by the grace with which he handles this roller coaster of a condition.

Despite every hurdle he has had to jump over, he has remained steadfastly Dan. He is himself. The vignettes Dan recounts about his experiences practicing medicine give an accurate glimpse into Dan as a person. He is kind beyond measure. He is unwaveringly loyal and devoted. He is a planner. He is tenacious. He is scrupulous. He is detail oriented, but he also appreciates the big picture. He has an uncanny sense of humor and a well-timed delivery of one-liners. He is self-deprecating and humble. He has a penchant for routine. He is curious, and his spirit for adventure is strong. His empathy is unmatched. He is a caring soul. He is a hopeless romantic. He is the boy I fell in love with, through and through. And with that on our side, our days are happy.

We live in a small community. Dan still has the opportunity to catch up with his patients from the practice, and they are genuinely overjoyed to see him. Without fail, Dan's first priority is to check on their status. "Did you follow up with that specialist?" "How are you doing with your blood pressure?" "Are you feeling well?" "Are you getting good care?" Patients still write him letters, ask about him, miss his care. He was Their Doctor. You can't unlearn that. Similarly, he will immediately launch into the role of Dad, of protector, of provider when he senses the need. It is innate. And, what's even better than me knowing this, is him realizing his sense of self remains.

Our days are dictated by his demeanor. They are enriched by episodes of his quick humor. One day, after he brushed his teeth, I handed him the bottle of mouthwash. He cradled it and with feigned emotion announced, "I'd like to thank the Academy . . ."

Our days are spontaneous and fun and full of love. We've been known to dance in the bathroom at two in the morning. He still looks at me like he's coming over to pick me up for a date.

Our days are filled with kindness. He sneaks bags of York peppermint patties into the shopping cart for me. He compliments everything:

"You're so pretty." (I had just come in from doing lawn work.)

"The kitchen looks great." (It didn't.)

"These scallops are so good!" (Those actually were quite good.)

He becomes the best host when people come over. Our guests are greeted with bags of candy, offers of drinks, his seat at the table.

Things get strained, however, when stressors emerge. Think of the biggest fears in your life, the ones that worry you and keep you up at night. Money? Health of your loved ones? Maintaining relationships? Loneliness? Safety? Planning for the future? Those big-ticket items are going to continue to be the ones that show up all the time. When these thoughts arise, don't be dismissive. Interact with compassion and, at all times, dignity. Listen actively. Trust that there is a reason behind the action and look for the root of the problem. Behavioral techniques relying on redirection are often not entirely successful because people with YOAD are aware of what is going on around them, and they often have a goal. As J. R. R. Tolkien so aptly pointed out, "Not all those who wander are lost." During these times, look for the qualities you've come to know and appreciate—they're in there. They might be hiding under depression, frustration, fear, anxiety. Tease them out. Believe they are there.

So what do you do for your loved one? What do I do for Dan, who has given of himself so selflessly to his family, his friends, his patients, and me? Anything. He deserves nothing less.

EPILOGUE

My name is Daniel Brown, which tells you nothing about me except that my parents were less than creative when it came time to fill out the birth certificate. Here are some of the details to fill in the gaps.

I love Monty Python. I think science is cool. I whistle around the house. I dated my wife for ten years before we got married. I really do want to help people. I have never fallen asleep in class. I love starting fires. I don't drive anymore. I prefer Jack and Coke or a nice whiskey. I had to apply to medical school twice. I started smoking when I was fourteen years old. My favorite color is gray. I never put the seat down. I try to get at least eight hours of sleep a night. I appreciate a tasty meatloaf. I could say the alphabet at two years old. I love mail. I still watch cartoons. My wife dresses me. I watch TV too often. I don't go to church as often as I should. My checkbook is balanced; my diet is not. I started golfing when I was eight years old and had not improved very much, so I gave it up. I have no accent. I don't play guitar very well. I'm a poor speaker but an excellent listener. I like change. I almost killed myself once. I've never seen Casablanca. I have been west of the Mississippi. I'm anal. Ten years from now I hope I'm on vacation. I am a Renaissance man. I love being a father. I have saved lives, *and my patients have died. The relationship that exists between doctor and patient is truly unique, and the aspect of medicine which I find most attractive. I believe in continuity of care, preventative medicine, and all the other catchphrases that have been used to describe family practice. The most important things in my life are my wife, my family, my friends, and a sense of humor. That's it. That is what it is all about. I felt that I was very good at what I did, but not at the expense of what I loved.*

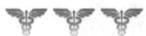

I hope people have realized the important things in their lives, too, because there is no part two. Be grateful.

FOR FURTHER READING

Bibliography

Altabakhi, Ibrahim W., and John W. Liang. "Gerstmann Syndrome." *Stat-Pearls*. StatPearls Publishing, 2023. https://www.ncbi.nlm.nih.gov/books/NBK519528/.

Alzheimer, A. "Uber einen eigenartigen schweren Erkrankungsprozess der Hirninde." *Neurologisches Centralblatt* 25 (1906): 1134.

Baas, Peter W., and Liang Qiang. "Tau: It's Not What You Think." *Trends in Cell Biology* 29, no. 6 (June 2019): 452–61. https://doi.org/10.1016/j.tcb.2019.02.007. PMID: 30929793; PMCID: PMC6527491.

Brothers, Holly M., Maya L. Gosztyla, and Stephen R. Robinson. "The Physiological Roles of Amyloid-β Peptide Hint at New Ways to Treat Alzheimer's Disease." *Frontiers in Aging Neuroscience* 10 (2018): 118. https://doi.org/10.3389/fnagi.2018.00118. PMID: 29922148; PMCID: PMC5996906.

Created Out of Mind. "Do I See What You See? A Film about Dementia, Disconnection, and Seeing the World Differently." Video, April 19, 2018. https://www.youtube.com/watch?v=jekW8Z93LMw.

Culpepper, Larry, Marwan N. Sabbagh, Cheryll Allen, Abimbola Farinde, Stephanie Joyce, M. David Rudd, and Soundarya Gowda. "Advanced Strategies to Identify and Manage Early Alzheimer's Disease in Clinical Practice." Webinar, March, 2023.

De Renzi, Ennio, and Pietro Faglioni. "Apraxia." *Handbook of Clinical and Experimental Neuropsychology*, pp. 421-440. Psychology Press, 2020.

Dickinson, James A. "Lesser-Spotted Zebras: Their Care and Feeding." *Canadian Family* Physician 62, no. 8 (2016): 620-621. PMID: 27521381; PMCID: PMC4982713.

Goldenberg, Georg. *Apraxia: The Cognitive Side of Motor Control*. Oxford: Oxford University Press, 2013.

Hendriks, Stevie, Kirsten Peetoom, Christian Bakker, Wiesje M. van der Flier, Janne M. Papma, Raymond Koopmans, Frans R. J. Verhey, et al. "Global Prevalence of Young-Onset Dementia." *JAMA Neurology* 78, no. 9 (July 19, 2021). https://doi.org/10.1001/jamaneurol.2021.2161. PMID: 34279544; PMCID: PMC8290331.

Henry, Maya L, and Maria Luisa Gorno-Tempini. "The Logopenic Variant of Primary Progressive Aphasia." *Current Opinion in Neurology* 23, no. 6 (December 2010): 633–37. https://doi.org/10.1097wco.0b013e32833fb93e. PMID: 20852419; PMCID: PMC3201824.

Kojovic, Maja, Carla Cordivari, and Kailash Bhatia. "Myoclonic Disorders: A Practical Approach for Diagnosis and Treatment." *Therapeutic Advances in Neurological Disorders* 4, no. 1 (January 2011): 47–62. https://doi.org/10.1177/1756285610395653. PMID: 21339907; PMCID: PMC3036960.

Kvello-Alme, Marte, Geir Bråthen, Linda R. White, and Sigrid Botne Sando. "Time to Diagnosis in Young Onset Alzheimer's Disease: A Population-Based Study from Central Norway." *Journal of Alzheimer's Disease* 82, no. 3 (2021): 965-974. https://doi.org/10.3233/JAD-210090. PMID: 34120901; PMCID: PMC8461696.

Llibre-Guerra, Jorge J., Leonardo Iaccarino, Dean Coble, Lauren Edwards, Yan Li, Eric McDade, Amelia Strom et al. "Longitudinal Clinical, Cognitive and Biomarker Profiles in Dominantly Inherited Versus Sporadic Early-Onset Alzheimer's Disease." *Brain Communications* 5, no. 6 (2023): fcad280.

Mendez, Mario F. "Early-Onset Alzheimer Disease and Its Variants." *CONTINUUM: Lifelong Learning in Neurology* 25, no. 1 (February 2019): 34–51. https://doi.org/10.1212/con.0000000000000687. PMID: 30707186; PMCID: PMC6538053.

Mendez, Mario F., Youssef I. Khattab, and Oleg Yerstein. "Clinical Screening for Posterior Cortical Atrophy." *Cognitive and Behavioral Neurology* 35, no. 2 (June 2022): 104–9. https://doi.org/10.1097/wnn.0000000000000297.

Mesulam, M-Marsel. "Slowly Progressive Aphasia without Generalized Dementia." *Annals of Neurology: Official Journal of the American Neurological Association and the Child Neurology Society* 11, no. 6 (1982): 592-598. https://doi.org/10.1002/ana.410110607.

O'Brien, Richard J., and Philip C. Wong. "Amyloid Precursor Protein Processing and Alzheimer's Disease." *Annual Review of Neuroscience* 34, no. 1 (2011): 185-204. https://doi.org/10.1146/annurev-neuro-061010-113613. PMID: 21456963; PMCID: PMC3174086.

Park, Jung E. "Apraxia: Review and Update." *Journal of Clinical Neurology* 13, no. 4 (2017): 317–324. https://doi.org/10.3988/jcn.2017.13.4.317. PMID: 29057628; PMCID: PMC5653618.

Rabinovici, Gil D. "Late-Onset Alzheimer Disease." *Continuum: Lifelong Learning in Neurology* 25, no. 1 (2019): 14–33. https://doi.org/10.1212/CON.0000000000000700. PMID: 30707185; PMCID: PMC6548536.

Schott, Jonathan M., and Sebastian J. Crutch. "Posterior Cortical Atrophy." *CONTINUUM: Lifelong Learning in Neurology* 25, no. 1 (February 2019): 52–75. https://doi.org/10.1212/con.0000000000000696. PMID: 30707187; PMCID: PMC6548537.

Tolkien, J.R.R. *The Fellowship of the Ring*. London: HarperCollins Publishers, 1991.

Van Erum, Jan, Debby Van Dam, and Peter Paul De Deyn. "Alzheimer's Disease: Neurotransmitters of the Sleep-Wake Cycle." *Neuroscience & Biobehavioral Reviews* 105 (October 2019): 72–80. https://doi.org/10.1016/j.neubiorev.2019.07.019.

Yang, Hyun Duk, Do Han Kim, Sang Bong Lee, and Linn Derg Young. "History of Alzheimer's Disease." *Dementia and Neurocognitive Disorders* 15, no. 4 (December 2016): 115. https://doi.org/10.12779 /dnd.2016.15.4.115. PMID: 30906352; PMCID: PMC6428020.

Online Resources

Alzheimer's Association: www.alz.org

Alzheimer's Research UK: www.alzheimersresearchuk.org

American Association of Neurological Surgeons: www.aans.org

The Cerebral Cortex: my.clevelandclinic.org/health/articles/23073-cere-bral-cortex

Identify Alzheimer's Disease: www.identifyalz.eu

Johns Hopkins Medicine: https://www.hopkinsmedicine.org/

Rare Dementia Support: www.raredementiasupport.org

ACKNOWLEDGMENTS

This book has been both a labor of love and a privilege to write. To see it through to completion is a dream come true. We would like to thank the following people, without whose help this project would not have been seen to fruition.

To our editor, Fred Levine—an expert in the judicious use of semicolons and wordsmith extraordinaire, you listened patiently, heard our wishes, and provided the guidance and vision we needed to say what we really wanted to say in a way that made sense. And to our designer, Susan Turner, and the rest of the team at Small Batch Books in Amherst, Massachusetts. Thanks for making this book real.

To Dan's patients, mentioned and not. This book came about because of you. Dan loved being a doctor and is deeply humbled that he was allowed to care for you. The tremendous responsibility and honor to treat patients with respect and dignity to the best of his ability are not lost on him. Thank you for trusting him enough to call him Doc.

To our Tufts crew: the Drays, the Karels, the Rosenzweigs, and the Turners. You keep our spirits high and buoy us with love, laughter, and memories. Thank you for traversing all over the country to be with us and for being constants in our lives since you were Jumbos with quirky nicknames and lots of hair.

To Steven and Naomi Stein. Thank you for being a consistent source of joy and love. We are grateful for your friendship and unwavering support of our entire family. Macallan and Fizgig forever!

To the FMA family, including the partners, the providers, the staff, and our awesome office manager, Stacy Corriveau, who was there from the beginning. (We are so lucky you quit that forklift-driving gig.) We love you and want you to know we appreciate all you have ever done for us and our family.

To our health-care network friends, especially Joe Weinstein, MD, and Morgan Smokler. Thank you for your fierce loyalty, your kindness, and for being the light in the darkness.

To Maureen's mom and dad, John and Dianne O'Neil, and her sisters, Jen and Karen. Your love and support over the years has been steadfast and immeasurable. We are beneficiaries of your countless good gestures and are incredibly appreciative.

To all of our wonderful neighbors, especially Donald and Terri Latimer, Guy Penha, the Rainho family, the Sousa family, Dolores and Joe Borges, the Nunes family, the Ferreiras, Debbie and Henry Zapasnik, and Krissy and Jamie Murphy. You are always there when we need you, and we are forever grateful.

To Becky Khayum, CCC-SLP, and Donna Bradley, PT, Maureen's confidants and sounding boards. Thank you both for being a gentle ear and a force of nature. Your support, wisdom, and friendship have been invaluable.

To Jerry Weisman, CPA, our trusted friend. We are immensely grateful for our decades-long friendship and your ability to find meaning and enjoyment in our banter. Thank you for your enthusiastic response to our project.

To Dan's medical team: Richard Popovic, MD, Sal Napoli, MD, Stacey Murray, NP, Nency Sangani, NP, and the team at

HopeHealth. Thanks for your compassionate care, for thinking outside the box, and for walking the path with us.

To Maureen's sister, Karen Cordischi, who was our enthusiastic first reader and privy to our project early on. She waited patiently and kept our confidence as we completed the manuscript. She listened intently to our progress during every "Friday-night dinner with Karen" and then, when we finally finished, took the day off to promptly read the copy in one sitting. Thank you for giving your thoughtful feedback and catching our punctuation errors, but even more importantly, for always being excited about the project and for confirming that it was well worth all of our time and effort. We cherished our time with you and were always grateful to have the opportunity to discuss the book. We deeply appreciate all you have done to support us in every way possible. You will always be our "Little Sista" and the kindest person we know.

And to our phenomenal kids. We understand and respect your privacy, but it's hard not to express the deep gratitude and enduring love we have for you. Thank you for embracing this project wholeheartedly, for being our cheerleaders at every turn, and for being just all-around good humans. Your boundless love and selfless nature are unmatched and will continue to be a constant source of joy and pride for both of us. Lorna has.

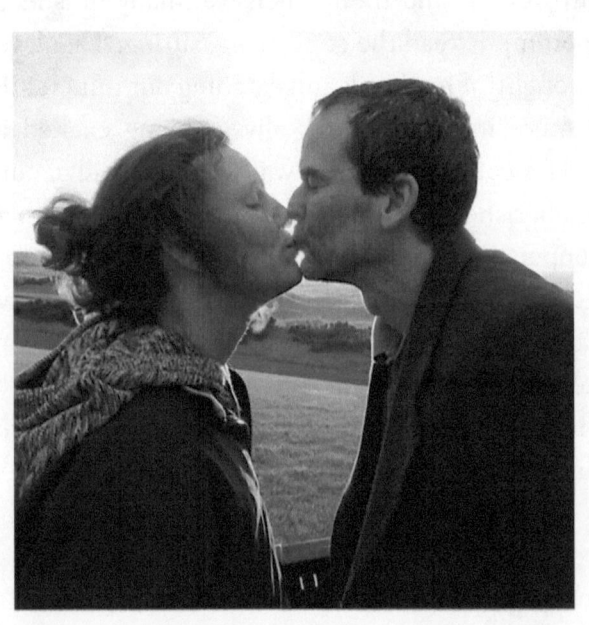

ABOUT THE AUTHORS

DAN BROWN worked as a family physician for twenty-eight years. He served the community in his capacity as a private practice physician, an adjunct faculty member with Brown University and Albany Medical Center, the medical director for a local skilled-nursing facility, and as the chief medical officer for a large health-care organization. Dan also served as a town doctor for two municipalities and mentored medical students in his practice.

MAUREEN BROWN is an occupational therapist who works as a care manager for clients diagnosed with neurodegenerative disorders, including Alzheimer's disease. Maureen assists by finding local resources, providing disease education, and supporting clients and their families.

DAN AND MAUREEN enjoyed hiking together, working in the yard, traveling, spending time with their kids, and going to their favorite date-night restaurant. Dan passed away in 2024, surrounded by his loving family.

www.ingramcontent.com/pod-product-compliance
Lightning Source LLC
Chambersburg PA
CBHW021654120626
46545CB00002B/862